JUL 2 7 2023

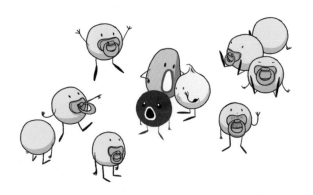

Down to the Bone

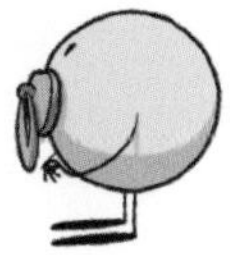

Library of Congress Cataloging-in-Publication Data

Names: Pioli, Catherine, 1982–2017, author.
Title: Down to the bone : a leukemia story / Catherine Pioli ; translated by J.T. Mahany.
Other titles: Globules et conséquences. English
Description: University Park, Pennsylvania : Graphic Mundi/Pennsylvania State University Press, [2022] | Original title: Globules et conséquences / Catherine Pioli. Editions Glénat, 2018.
Summary: "A narrative, in graphic novel format, of the author's life and experiences as a leukemia patient"—Provided by publisher.
Identifiers: LCCN 2022013181 | ISBN 9781637790342 (hardback ; alk. paper)
Subjects: MESH: Pioli, Catherine, 1982–2017. | Precursor Cell Lymphoblastic Leukemia-Lymphoma | France | Personal Narrative | Graphic Novel
Classification: LCC RC643 | NLM WH 17 | DDC 616.99/419—dc23/eng/20220330
LC record available at https://lccn.loc.gov/2022013181

Printed in China
Published by The Pennsylvania State University Press,
University Park, PA 16802-1003

Graphic Mundi is an imprint of The Pennsylvania State University.

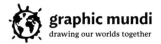

graphic mundi
drawing our worlds together

Translated by J.T. Mahany
Supplemental lettering by Indigo Kelleigh

Original Title: Globules et Conséquences
Author: Catherine Pioli

The Pennsylvania State University Press is a member of the Association of University Presses.

It is the policy of The Pennsylvania State University Press to use acid-free paper. Publications on uncoated stock satisfy the minimum requirements of American National Standard for Information Sciences—Permanence of Paper for Printed Library Material, ANSI Z39.48–1992.

Catherine Pioli

Down to the Bone

A Leukemia Story

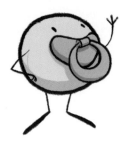

Translated by J.T. Mahany

graphic mundi

SHORT PROLOGUE
Corsica

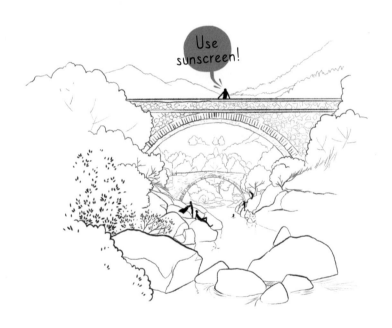

I grew up in a small town in Corsica. My twin sister, Emmanuelle, my younger brother, Gabriel, and I spent our free time outside, in nature. We romped around pretty much everywhere, building forts and the like. I don't think there's anything better for a healthy, happy childhood.

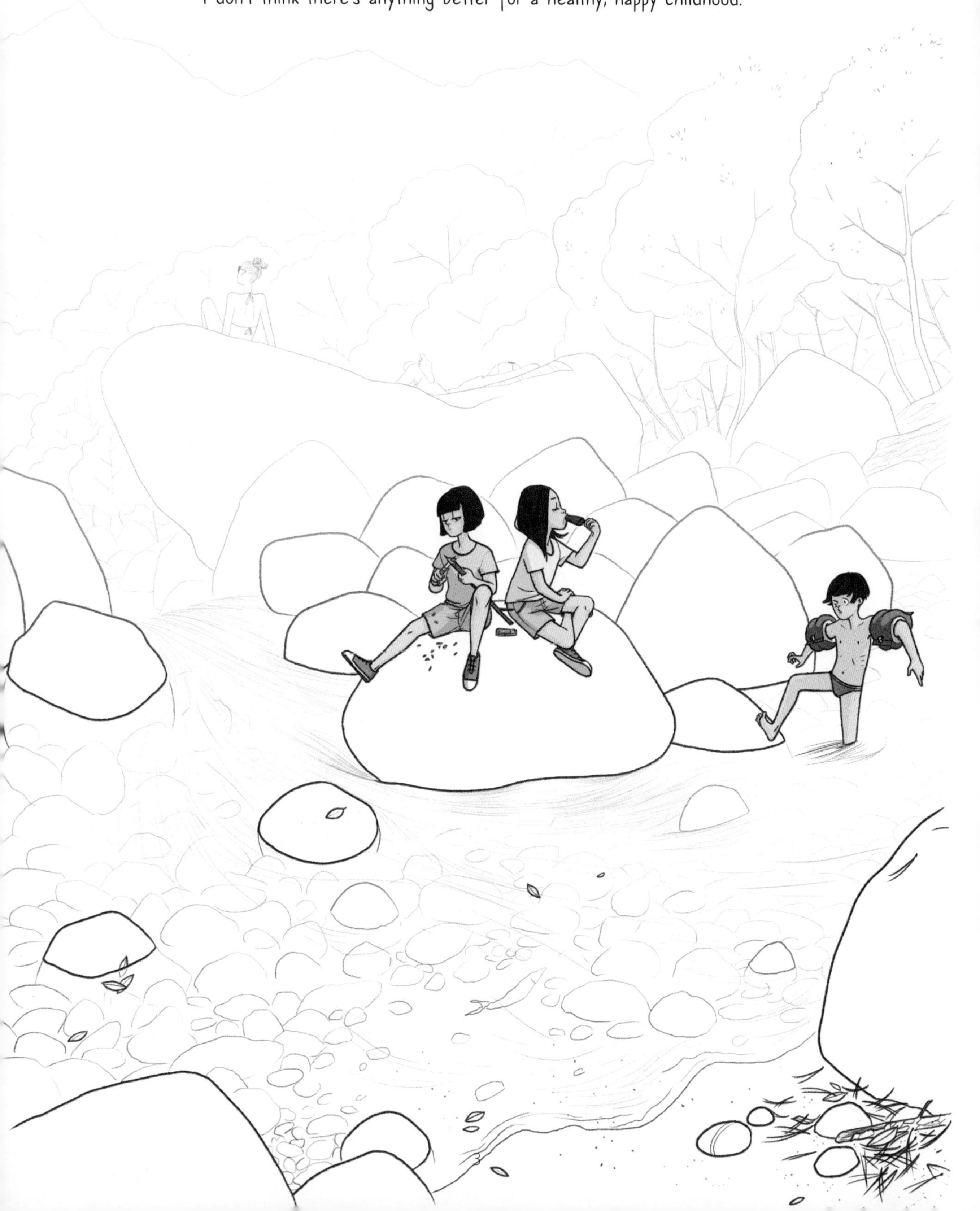

We each had a little pocket knife, bought by our father at the village's annual fair.
We nicked some matches from the kitchen drawer and *zip*! Off to the woods we went!

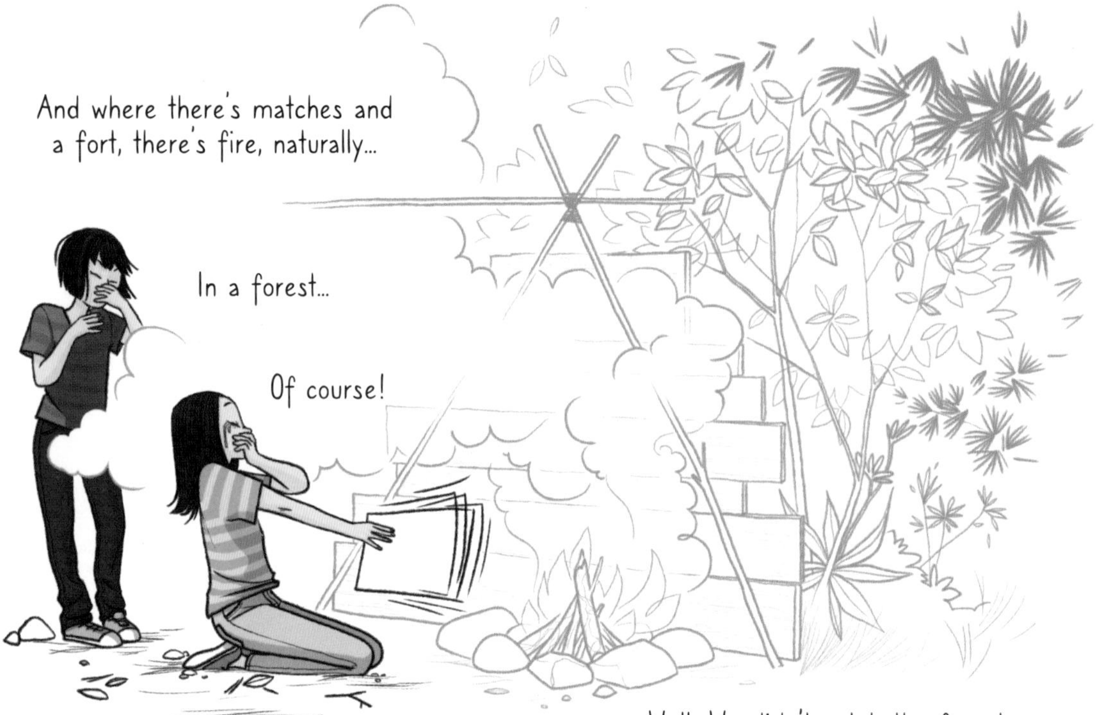
And where there's matches and a fort, there's fire, naturally...
In a forest...
Of course!

Well. We didn't catch the forest or our hair on fire, luckily. But we had plenty of other good ideas in the same vein...

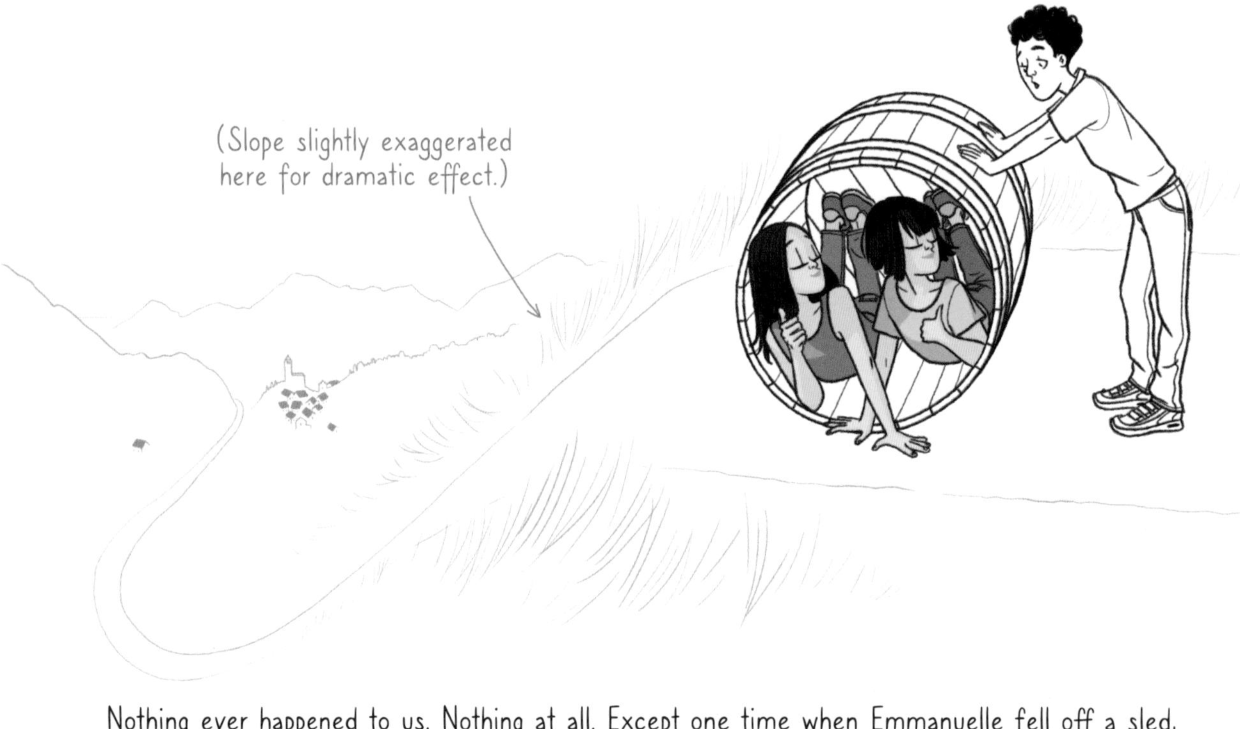
(Slope slightly exaggerated here for dramatic effect.)

Nothing ever happened to us. Nothing at all. Except one time when Emmanuelle fell off a sled, passed out, and had to spend the night in the hospital. But besides that, no sprains, fractures, viruses, allergies, or cavities (except Emmanuelle, again, who had her first one at age 33).

In short, I had always been used to my body
never giving me any problems and always
being in perfect health. I trusted it completely.
Broken bones were something friends got.

Lucky youuu!
BISOUS!
Remets toi vite!

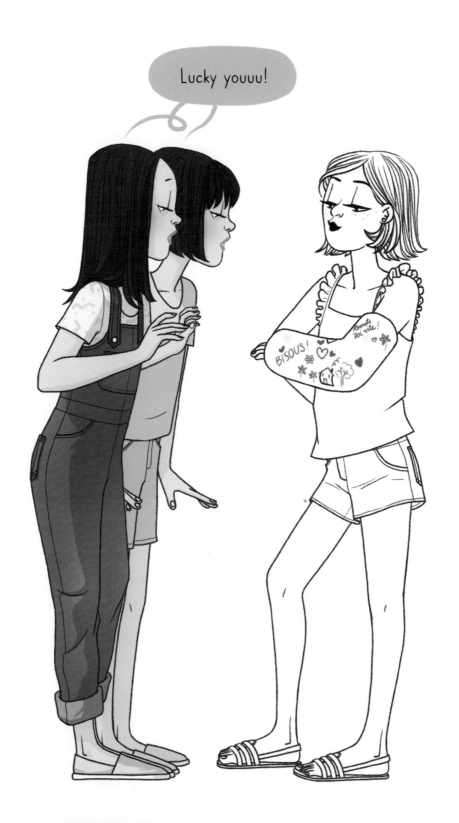

SUMMER/AUTUMN

Paris

Ow!

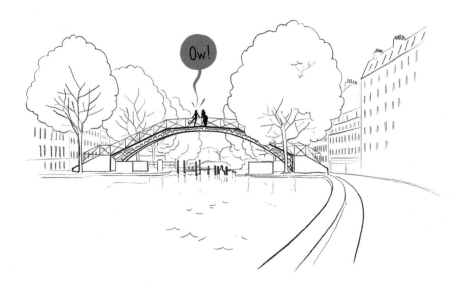

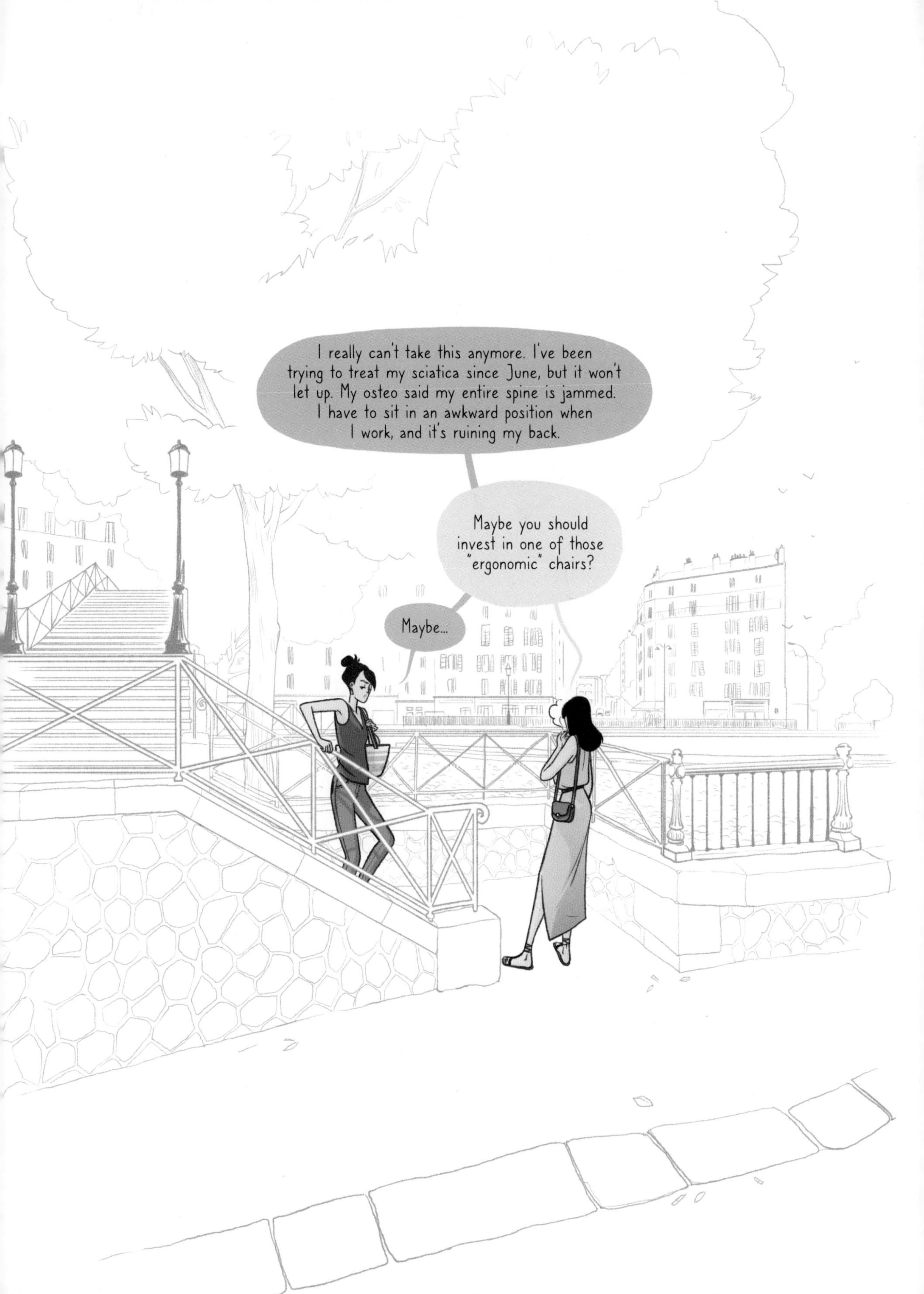
I really can't take this anymore. I've been trying to treat my sciatica since June, but it won't let up. My osteo said my entire spine is jammed. I have to sit in an awkward position when I work, and it's ruining my back.
Maybe you should invest in one of those "ergonomic" chairs?
Maybe...

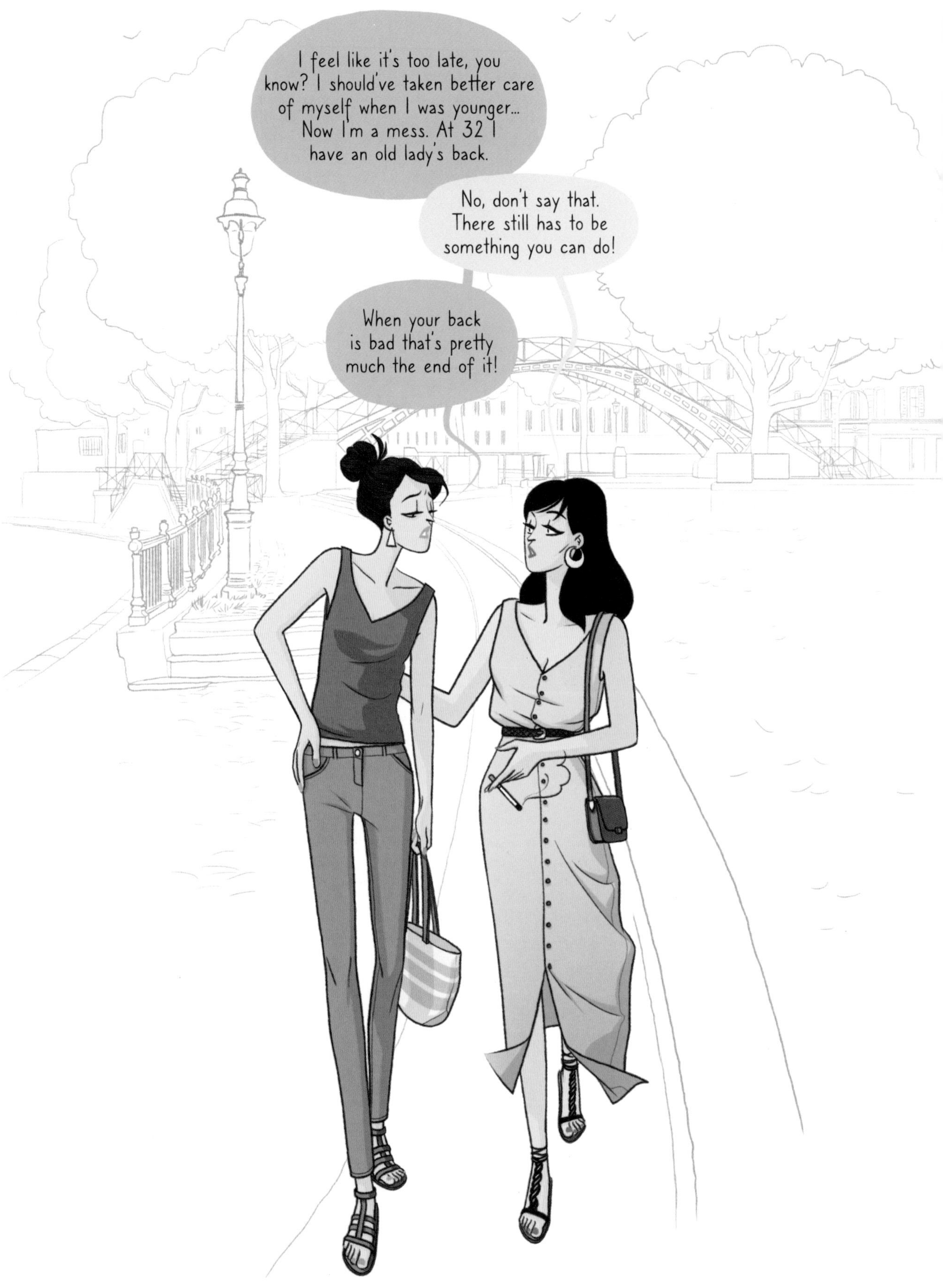
I feel like it's too late, you know? I should've taken better care of myself when I was younger... Now I'm a mess. At 32 I have an old lady's back.
No, don't say that. There still has to be something you can do!
When your back is bad that's pretty much the end of it!

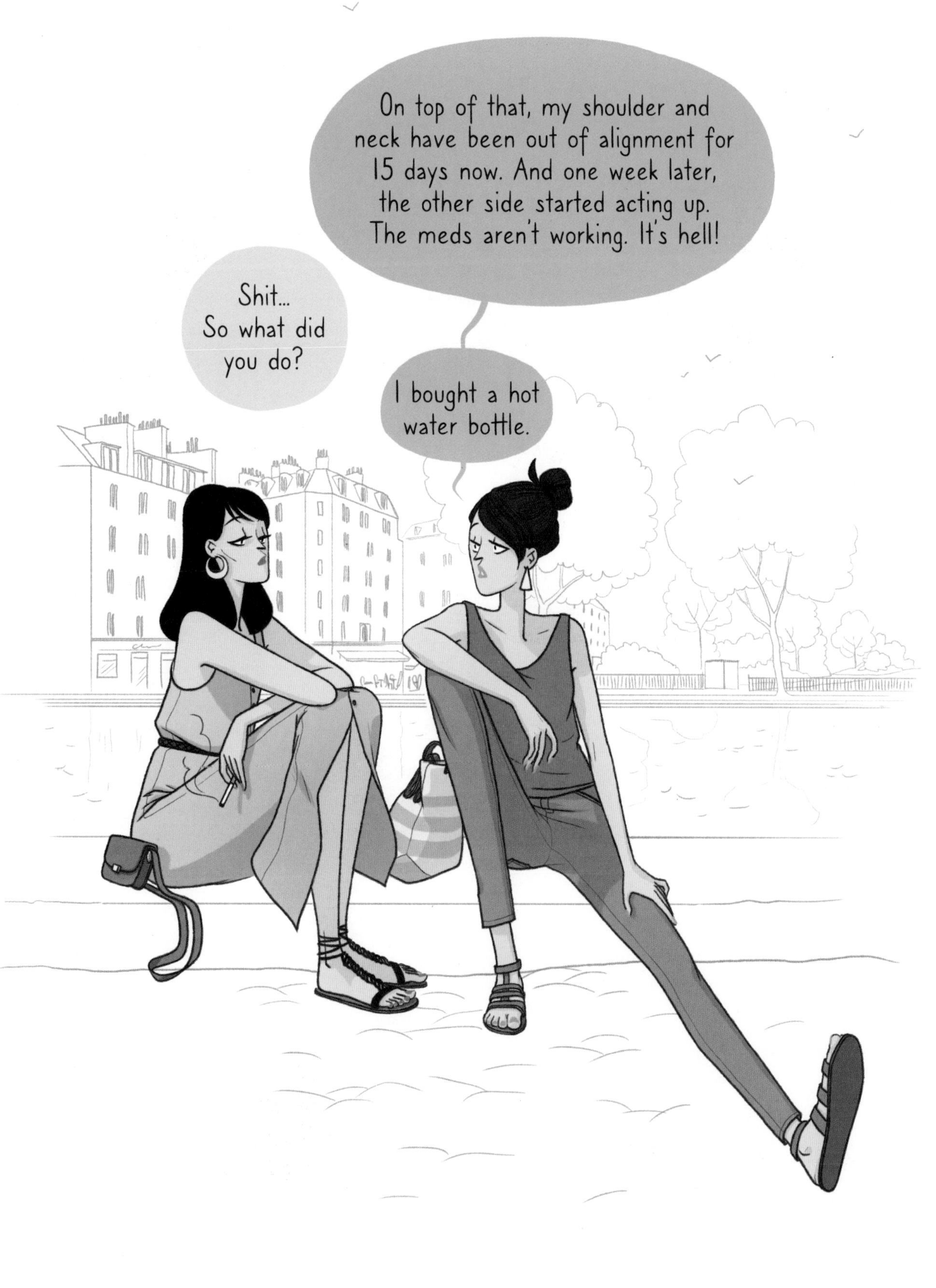
On top of that, my shoulder and neck have been out of alignment for 15 days now. And one week later, the other side started acting up. The meds aren't working. It's hell!
Shit... So what did you do?
I bought a hot water bottle.

FOR GREAT PAINS, GREAT REMEDIES

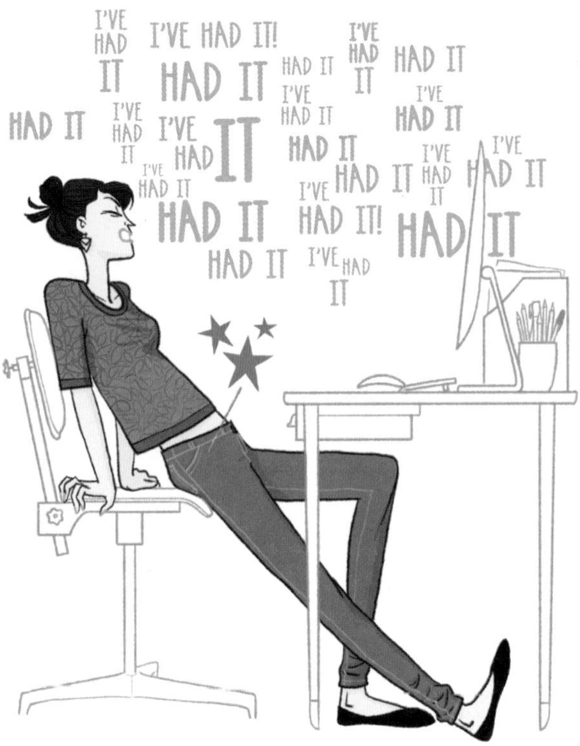
I'VE HAD IT I'VE HAD IT! I'VE HAD IT HAD IT HAD IT HAD IT HAD IT I'VE HAD IT I'VE HAD IT HAD IT I'VE HAD IT I'VE HAD IT HAD IT I'VE HAD IT I'VE HAD IT I'VE HAD IT HAD IT HAD IT I'VE HAD IT I'VE HAD IT HAD IT I'VE HAD IT HAD IT! HAD IT HAD IT I'VE HAD IT

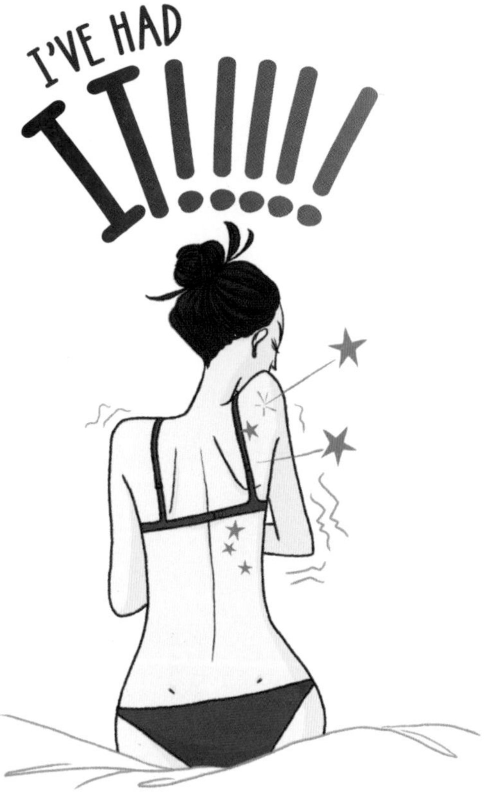
I'VE HAD IT!!!!!!

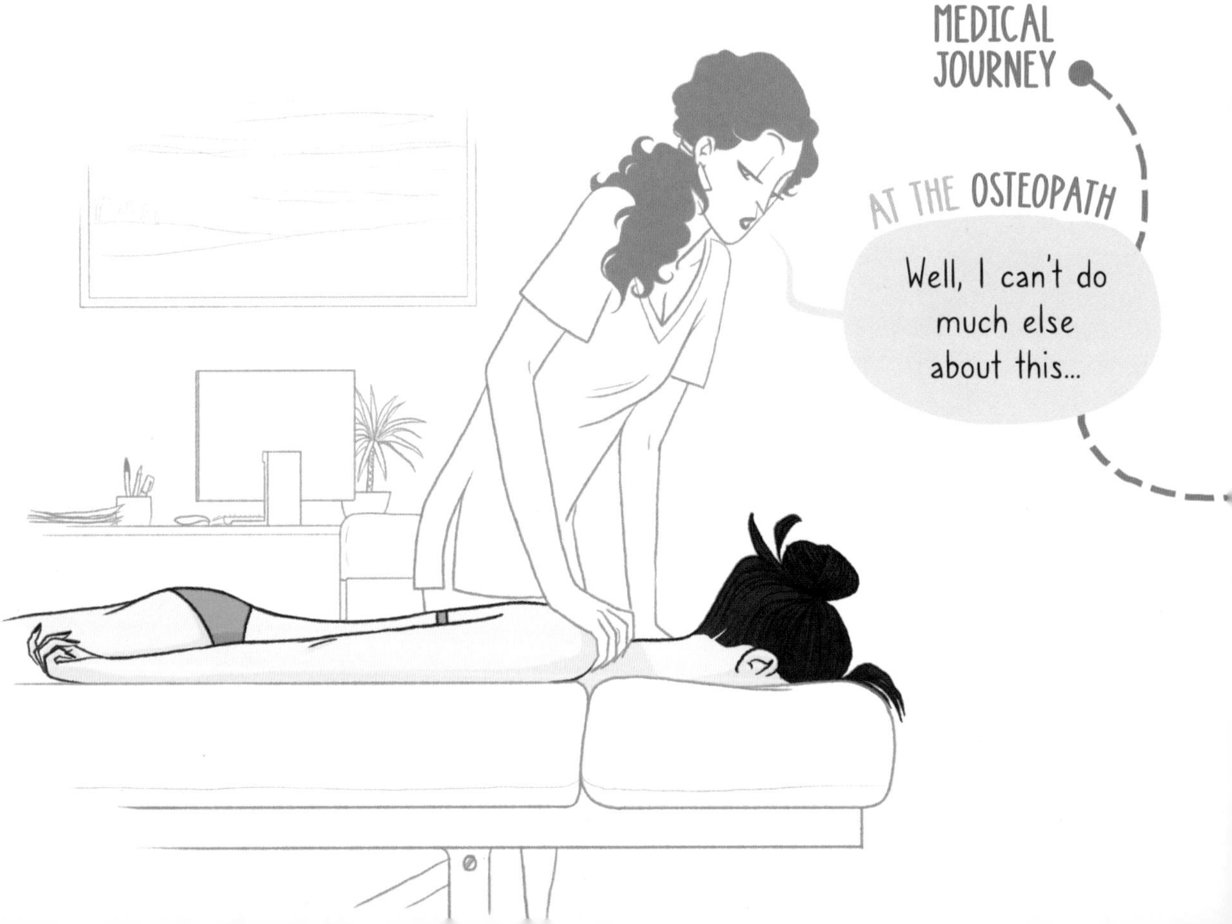
MEDICAL JOURNEY
AT THE OSTEOPATH
Well, I can't do much else about this...

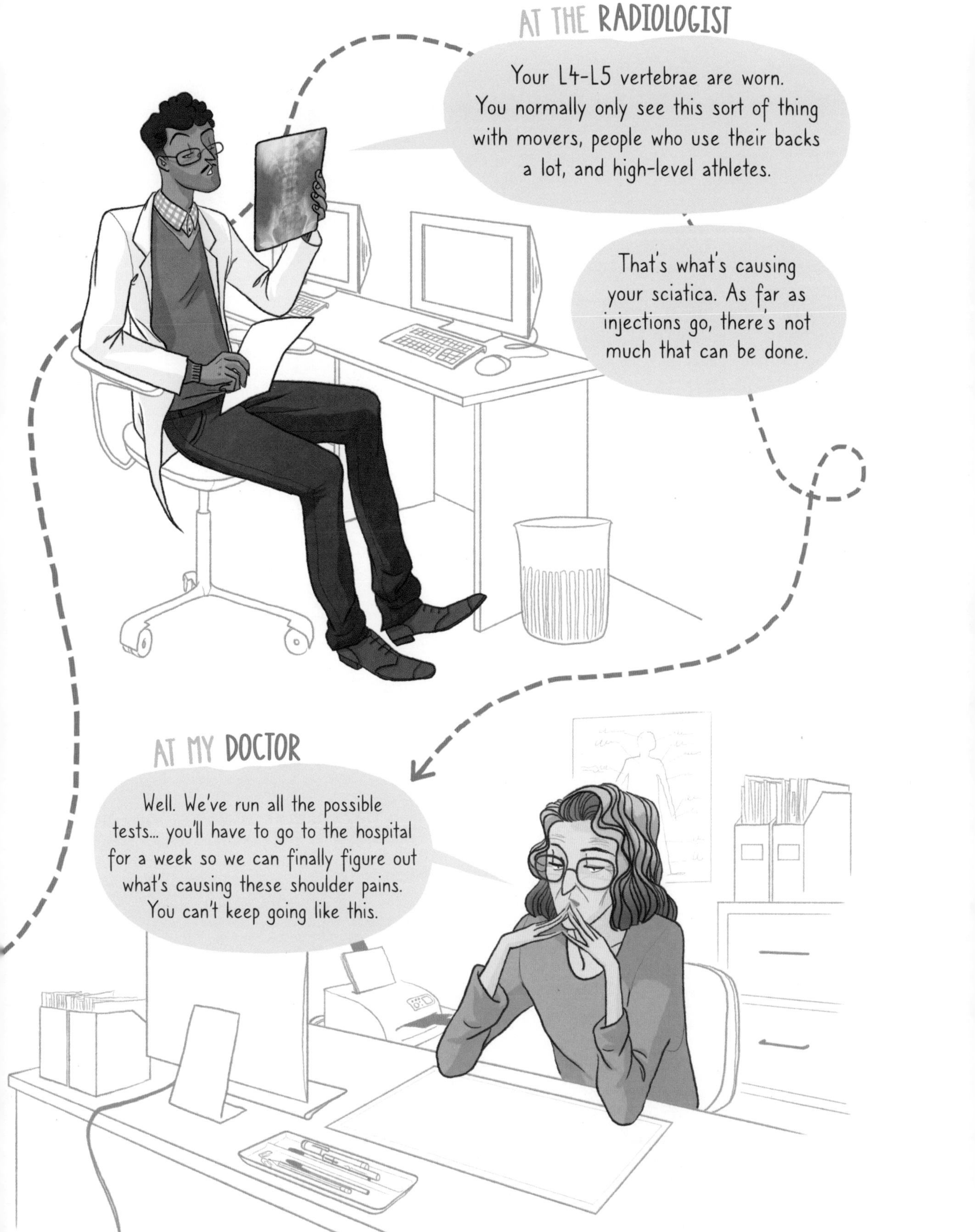
AT THE RADIOLOGIST
Your L4-L5 vertebrae are worn. You normally only see this sort of thing with movers, people who use their backs a lot, and high-level athletes.
That's what's causing your sciatica. As far as injections go, there's not much that can be done.
AT MY DOCTOR
Well. We've run all the possible tests... you'll have to go to the hospital for a week so we can finally figure out what's causing these shoulder pains. You can't keep going like this.

END OF NOVEMBER

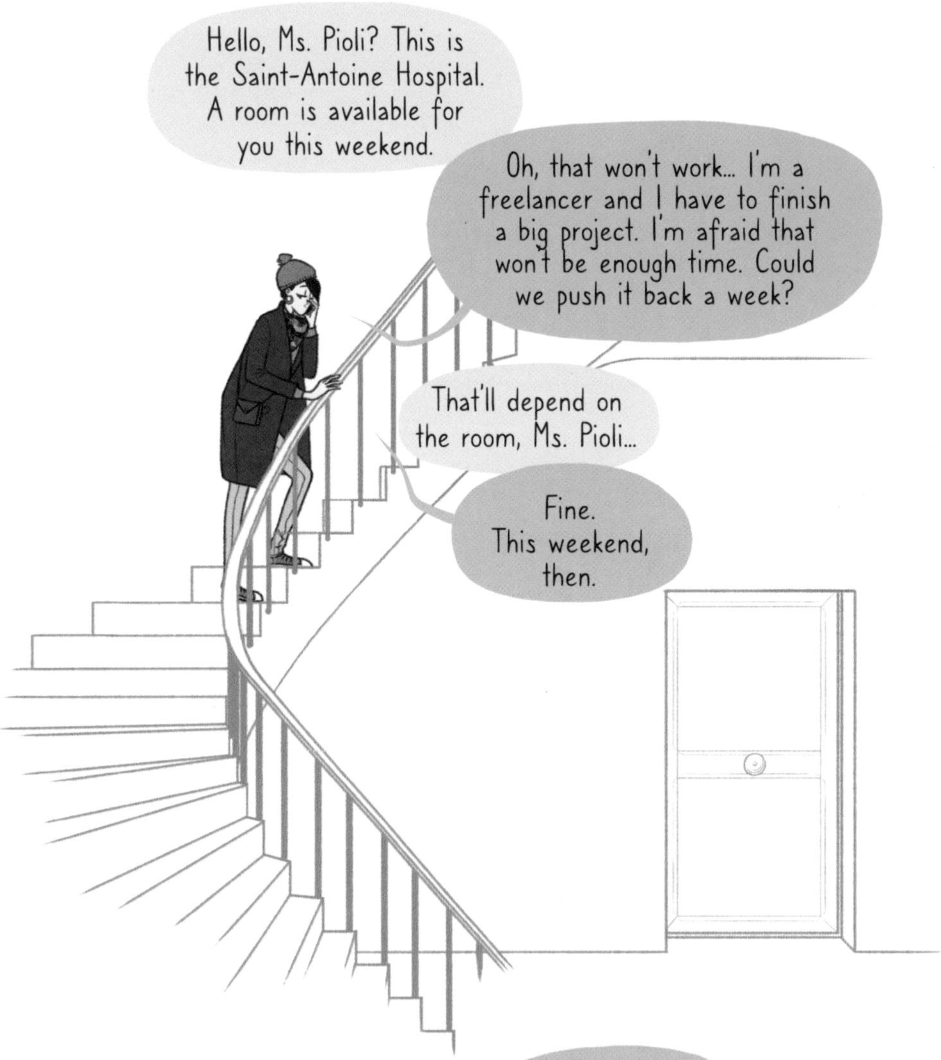

Hello, Ms. Pioli? This is the Saint-Antoine Hospital. A room is available for you this weekend.
Oh, that won't work... I'm a freelancer and I have to finish a big project. I'm afraid that won't be enough time. Could we push it back a week?
That'll depend on the room, Ms. Pioli...
Fine. This weekend, then.

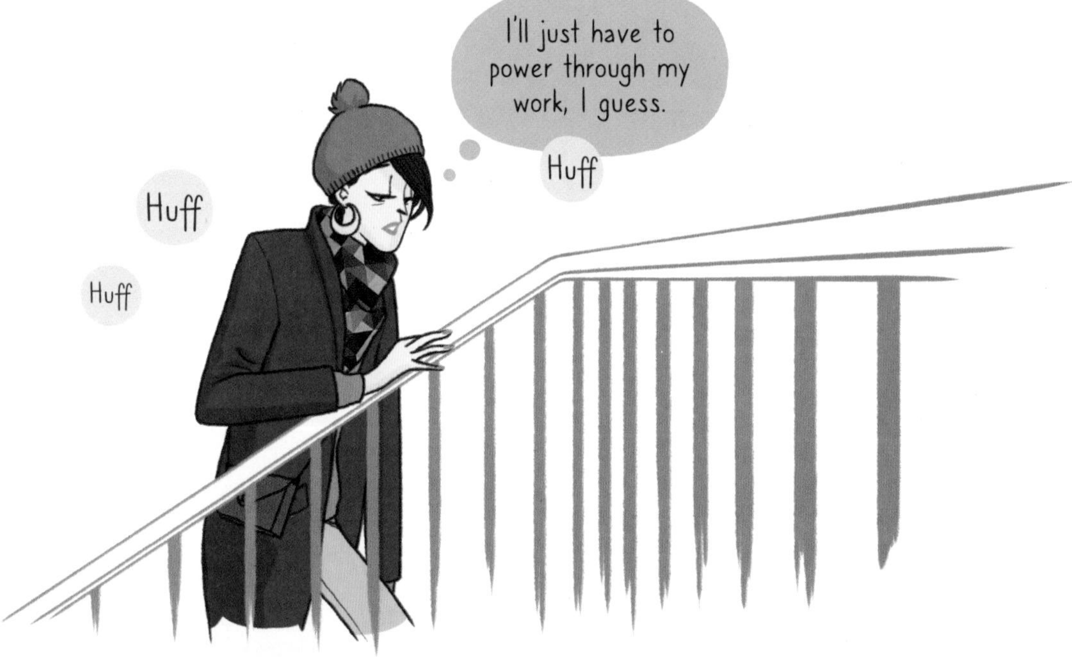

I'll just have to power through my work, I guess.
Huff
Huff
Huff

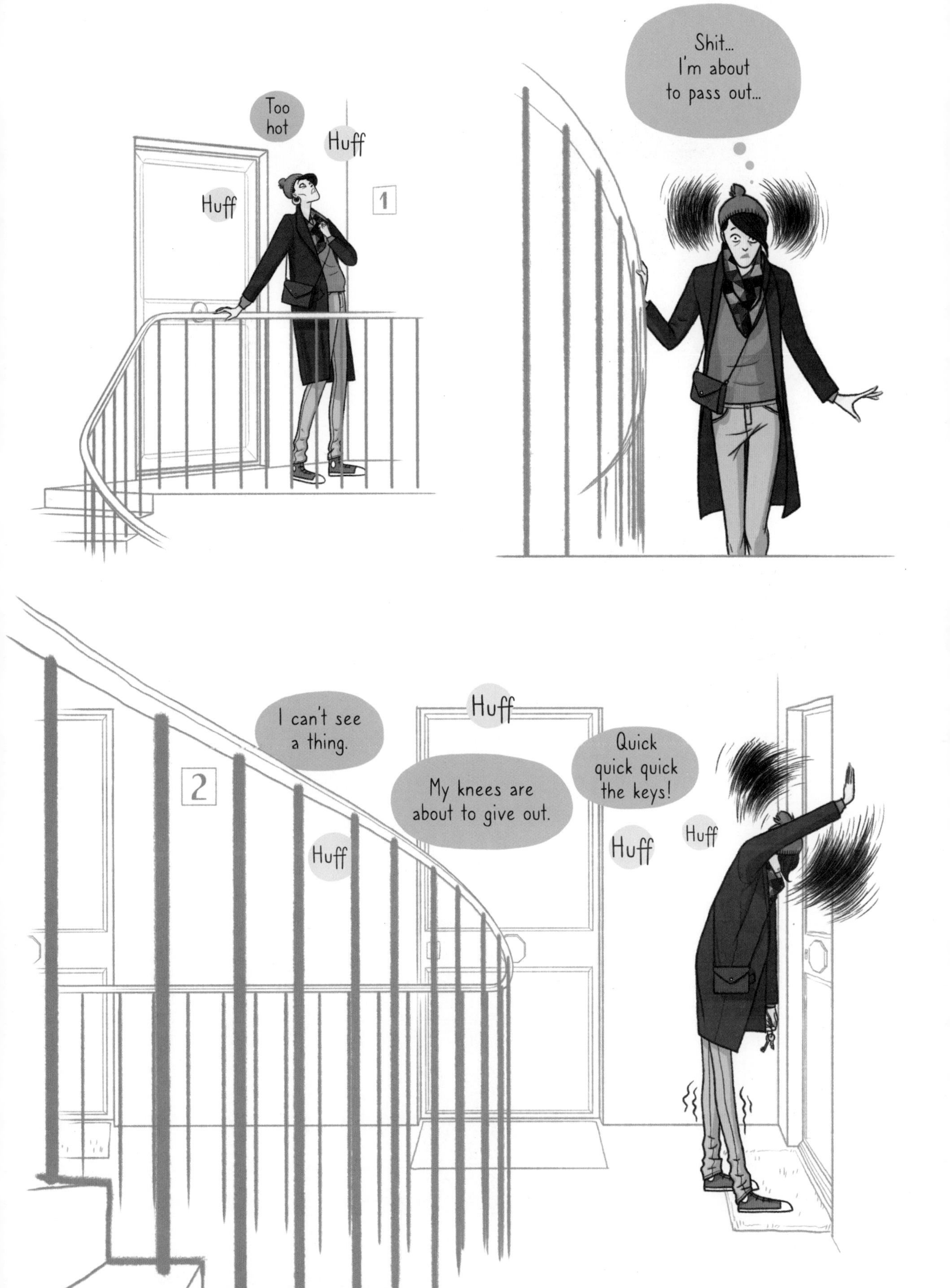
Too hot
Huff
Huff
Shit... I'm about to pass out...
I can't see a thing.
Huff
My knees are about to give out.
Huff
Quick quick quick the keys!
Huff
Huff

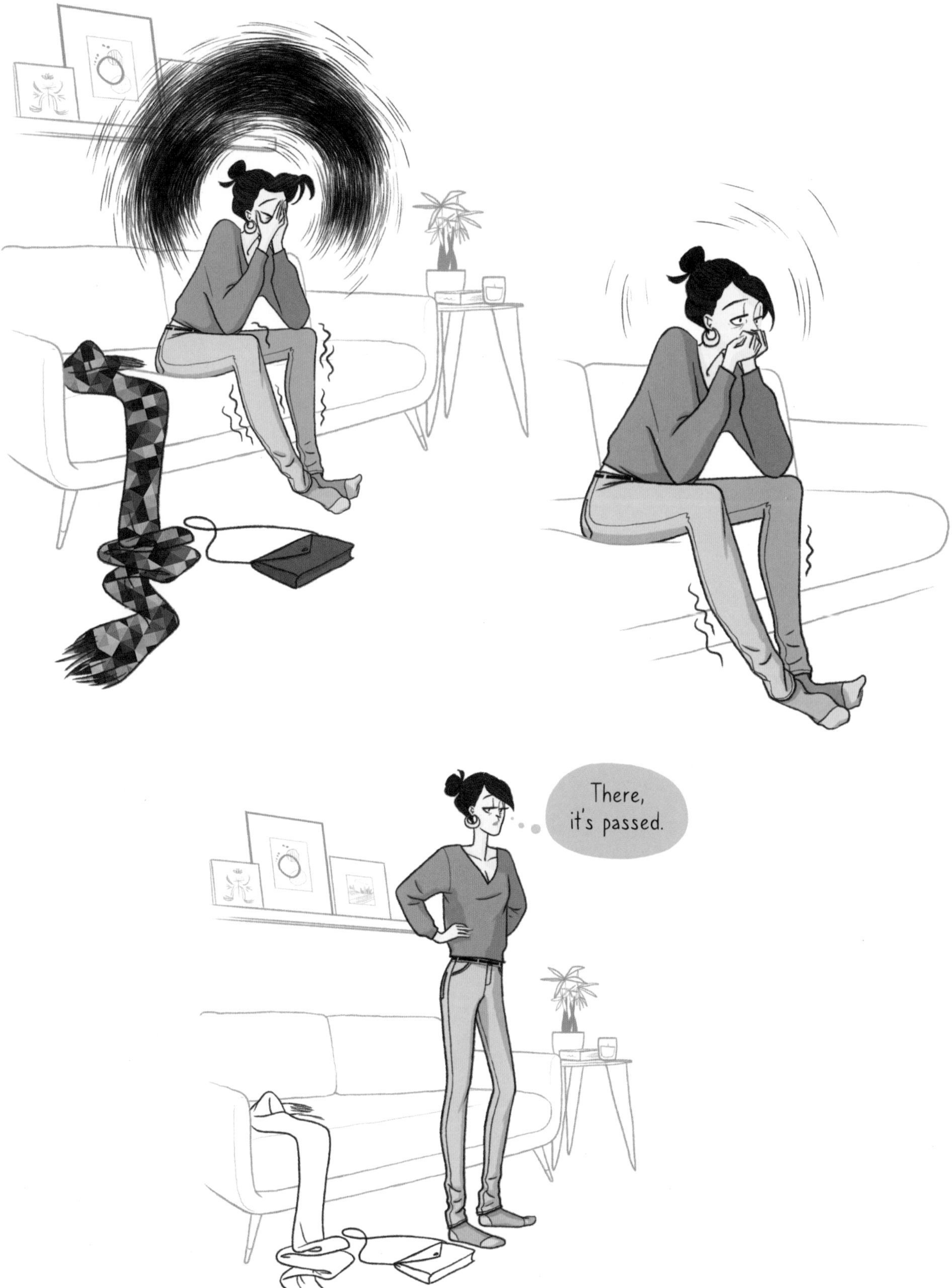
There, it's passed.

Ahhhhh fuck!

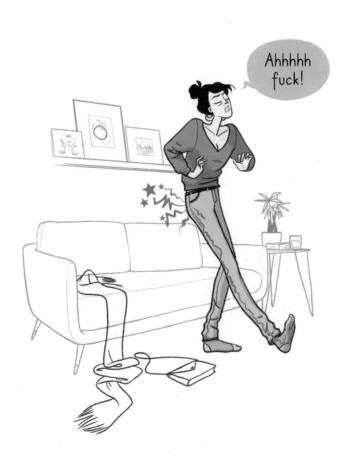

THE HOSPITAL

December 1st, 2 p.m.—On my way to the Saint-Antoine Hospital, Rheumatology Department

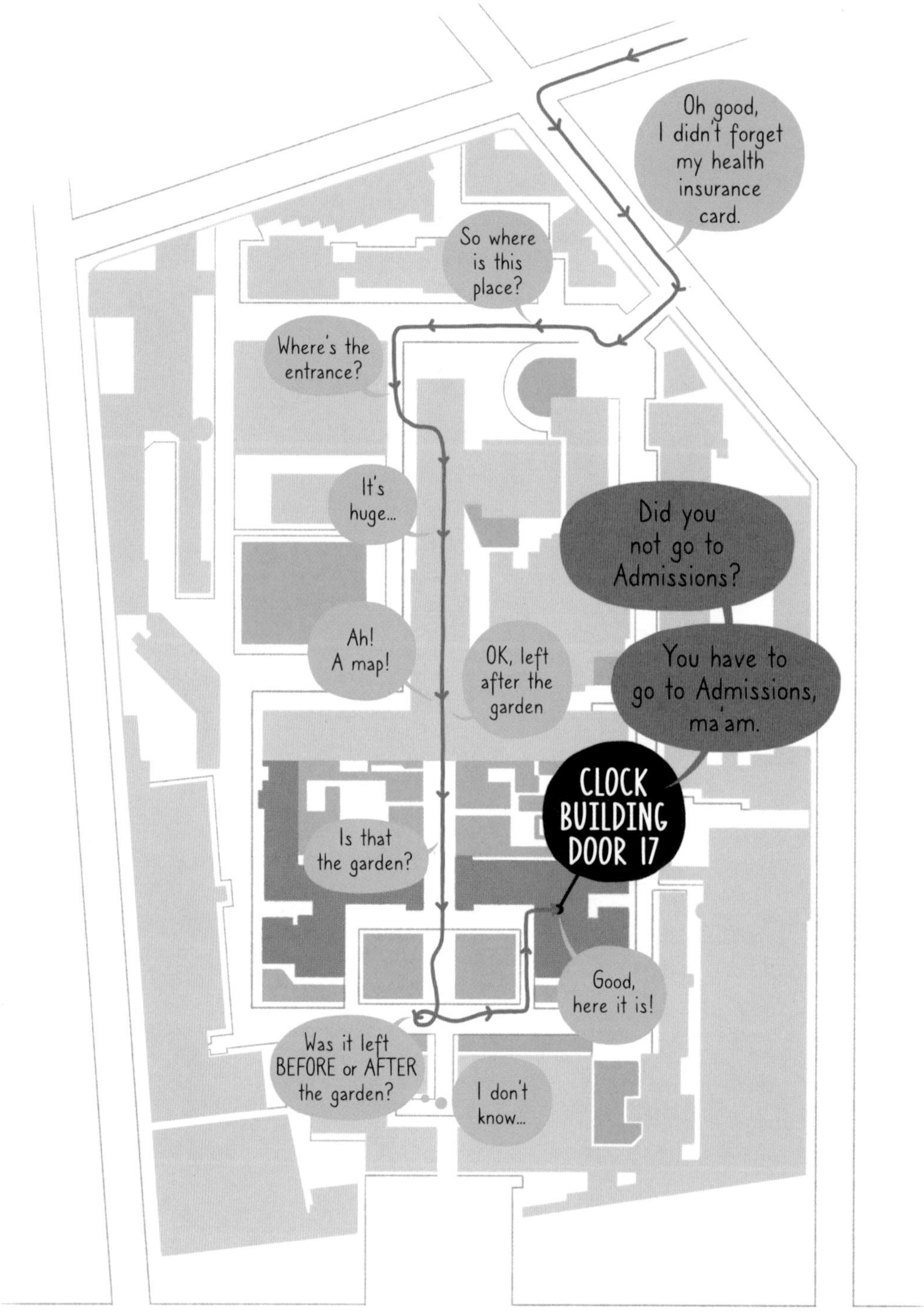

Oh good, I didn't forget my health insurance card.
So where is this place?
Where's the entrance?
It's huge...
Ah! A map!
OK, left after the garden
Is that the garden?
Was it left BEFORE or AFTER the garden?
I don't know...
Good, here it is!
CLOCK BUILDING DOOR 17
Did you not go to Admissions?
You have to go to Admissions, ma'am.

They didn't tell me much about the plan for the week.
All we did today was draw blood and measure vitals!

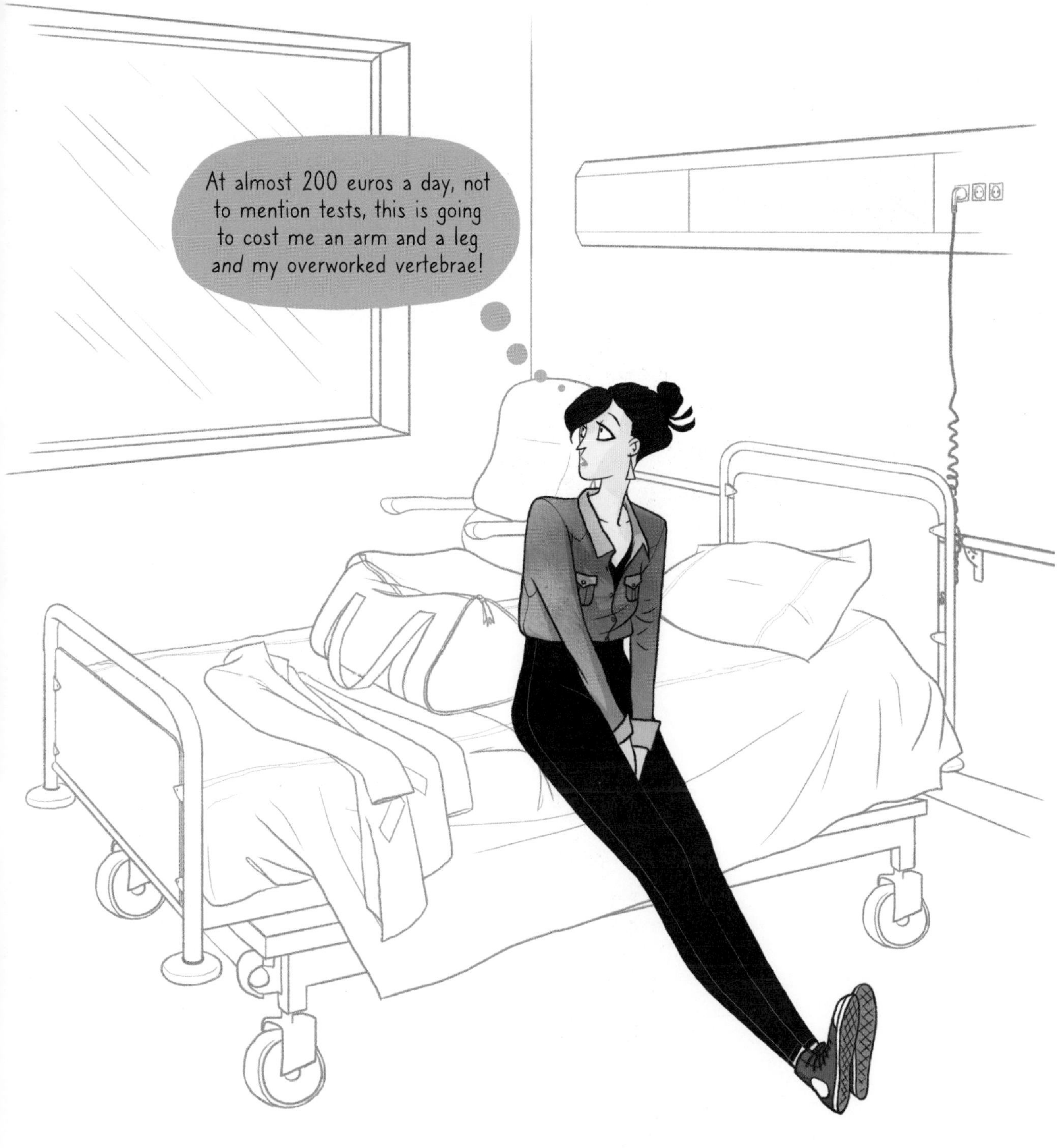
At almost 200 euros a day, not to mention tests, this is going to cost me an arm and a leg *and* my overworked vertebrae!

And finally at the end of the day, a group of doctors show up
with my test results. And they're wearing masks...

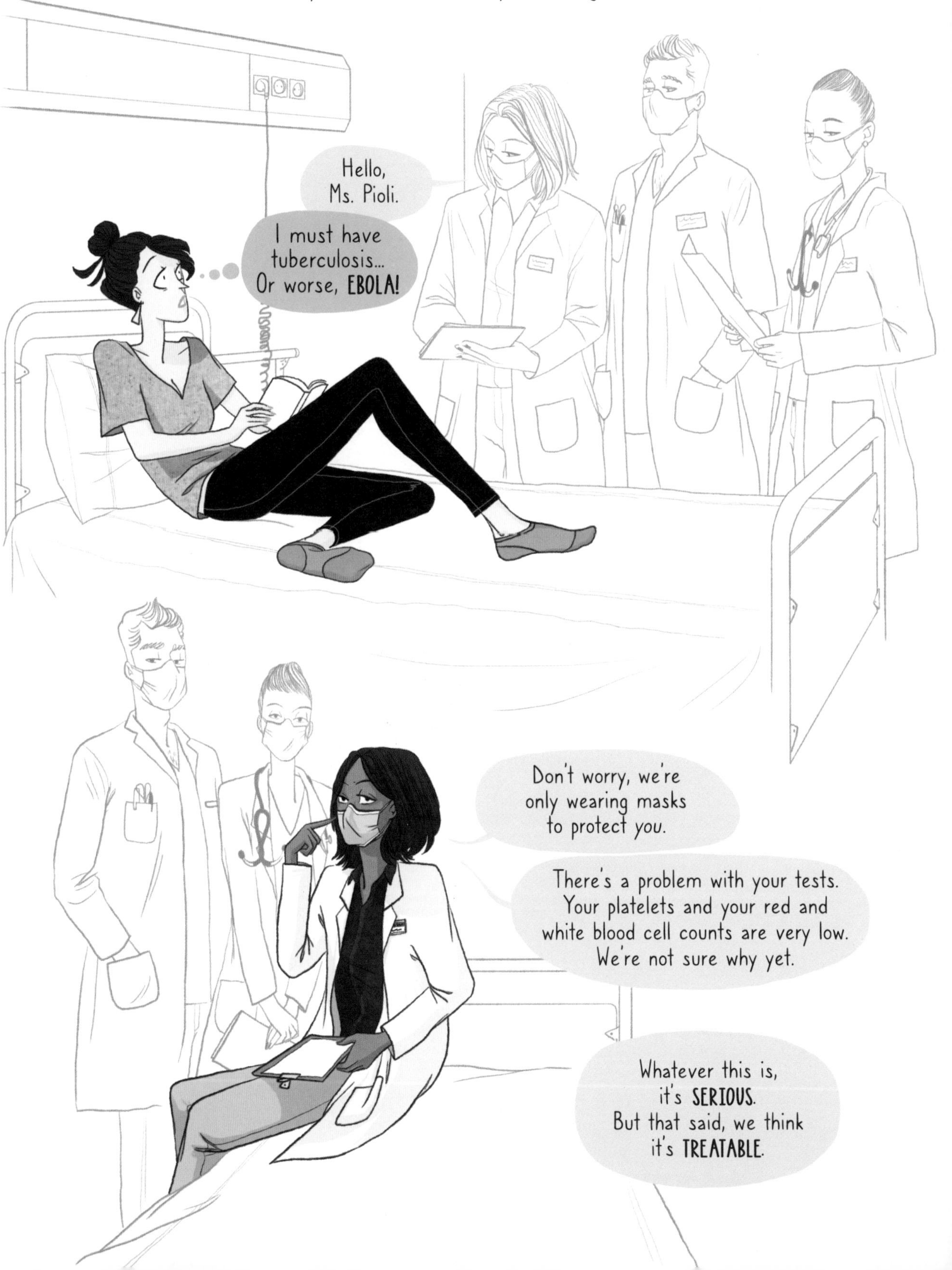
Hello, Ms. Pioli.
I must have tuberculosis... Or worse, **EBOLA!**
Don't worry, we're only wearing masks to protect *you*.
There's a problem with your tests. Your platelets and your red and white blood cell counts are very low. We're not sure why yet.
Whatever this is, it's **SERIOUS**. But that said, we think it's **TREATABLE**.

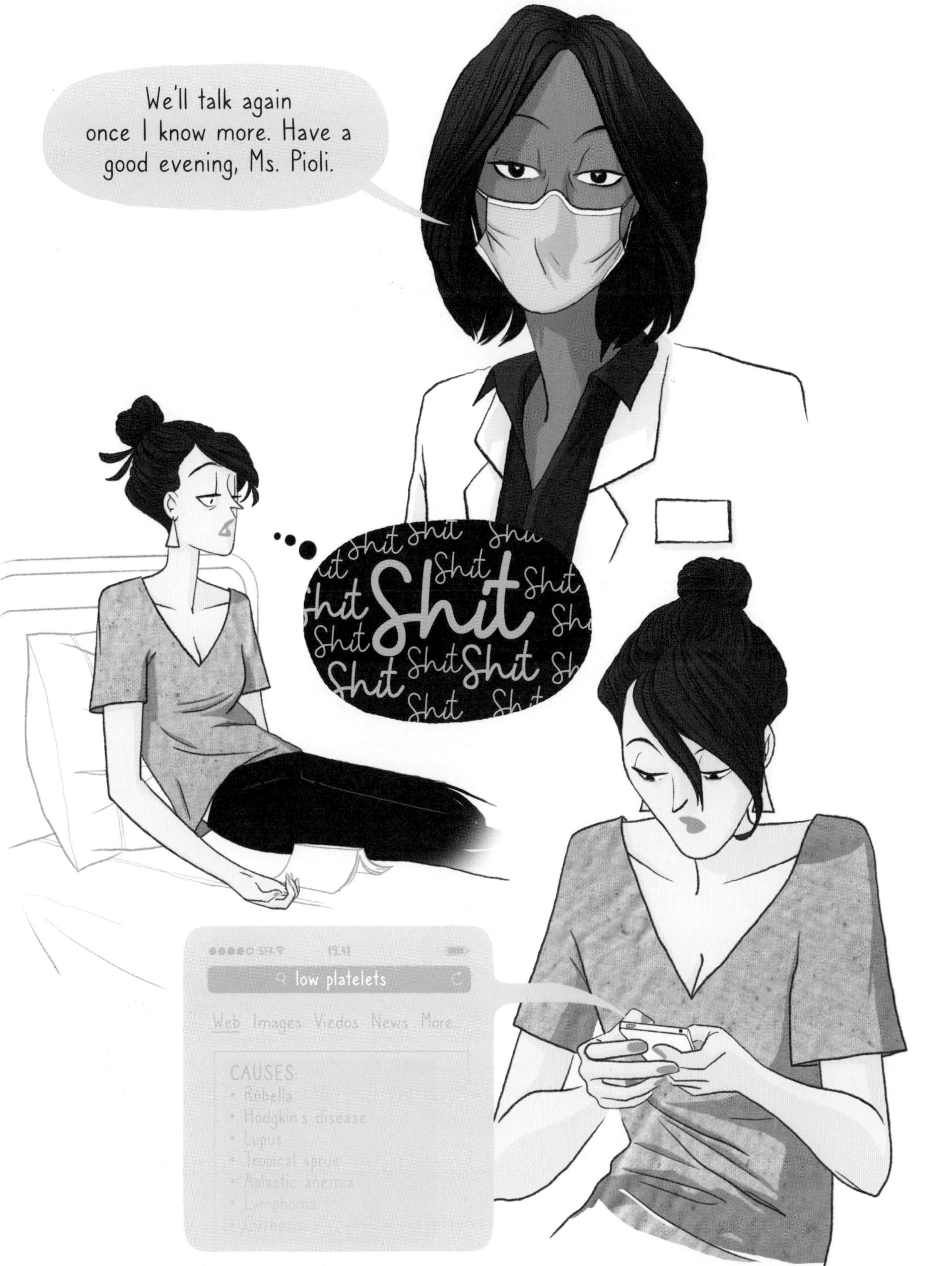
We'll talk again once I know more. Have a good evening, Ms. Pioli.
Shit Shit Shit Shit Shit Shit Shit Shit Shit Shit
SFR 19:48
low platelets
Web Images Viedos News More...
CAUSES:
• Rubella
• Hodgkin's disease
• Lupus
• Tropical sprue
• Aplastic anemia
• Lymphoma
• Cirrhosis

Note to self: don't use the internet to self-diagnose.
Everyone knows this, but we do it anyway.

GOLD MEDAL

It could have been anything, but the next day, I hadn't expected to win first prize.

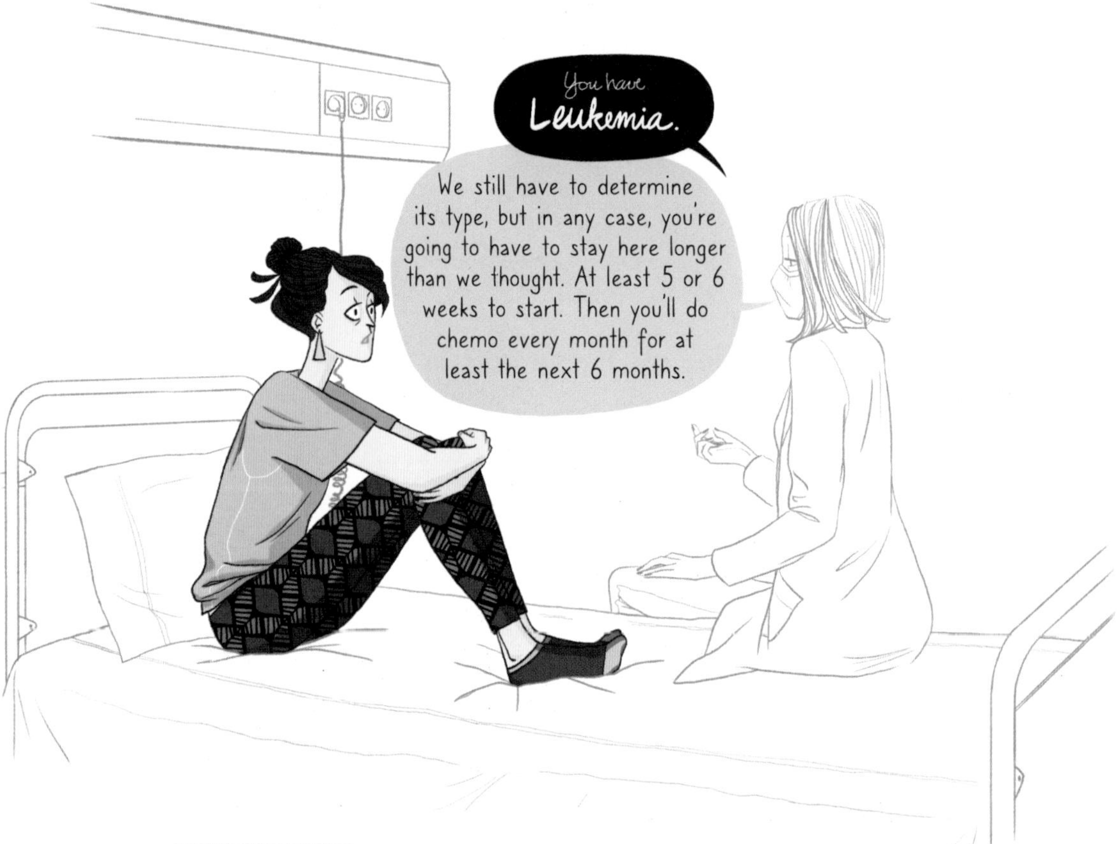
You have Leukemia.
We still have to determine its type, but in any case, you're going to have to stay here longer than we thought. At least 5 or 6 weeks to start. Then you'll do chemo every month for at least the next 6 months.

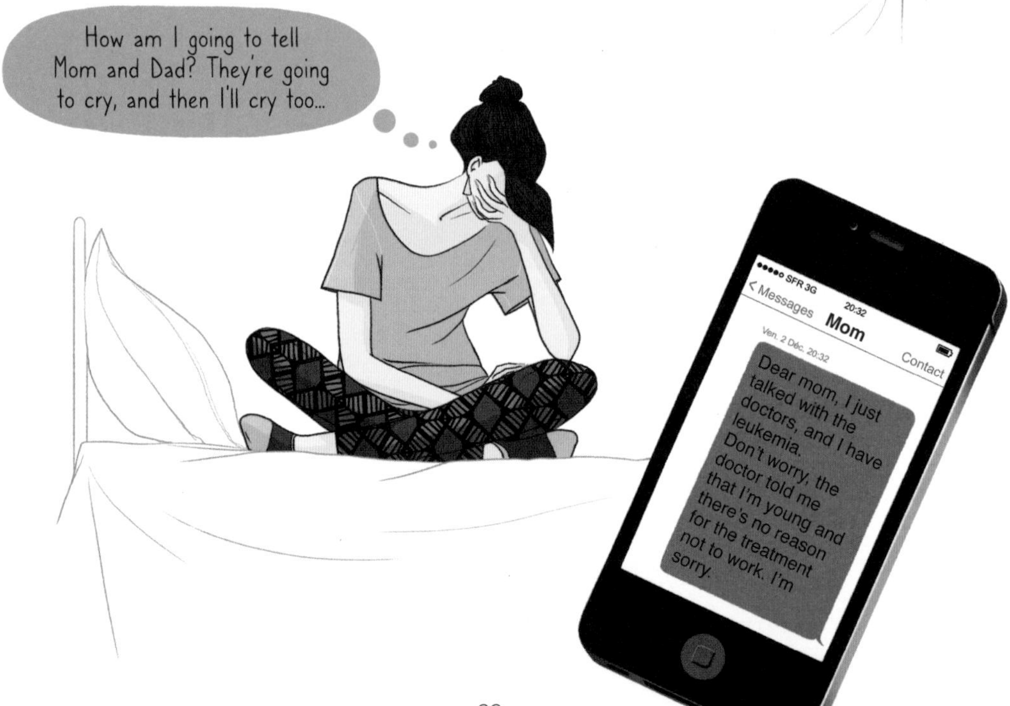
How am I going to tell Mom and Dad? They're going to cry, and then I'll cry too...
SFR 3G
20:32
< Messages
Mom
Contact
Ven. 2 Déc. 20:32
Dear mom, I just talked with the doctors, and I have leukemia. Don't worry, the doctor told me that I'm young and there's no reason for the treatment not to work. I'm sorry.

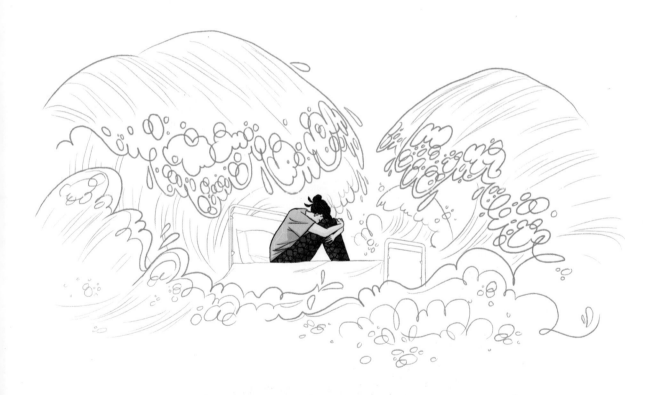

The next morning, I have to be transferred to the Hematology Department.

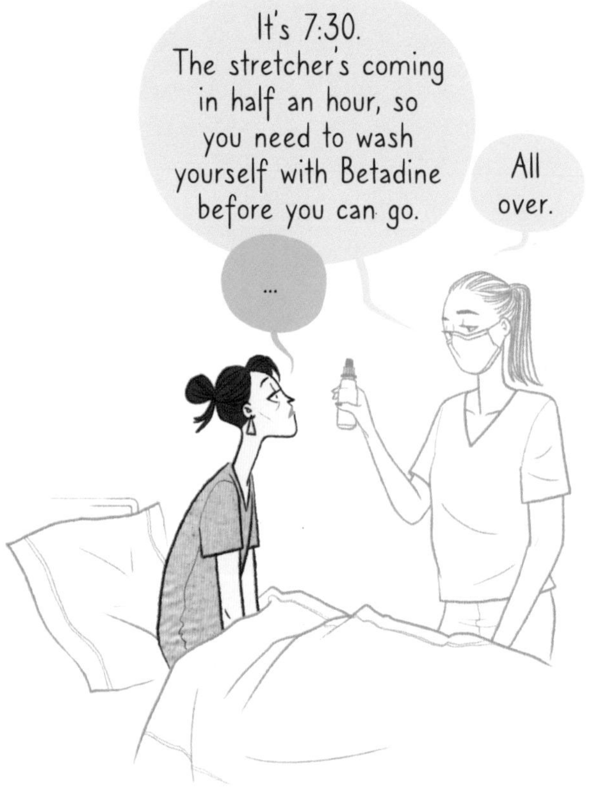
It's 7:30. The stretcher's coming in half an hour, so you need to wash yourself with Betadine before you can go.
...
All over.

I still don't understand what's happening. I feel dazed and passive. Like a walking potted plant.

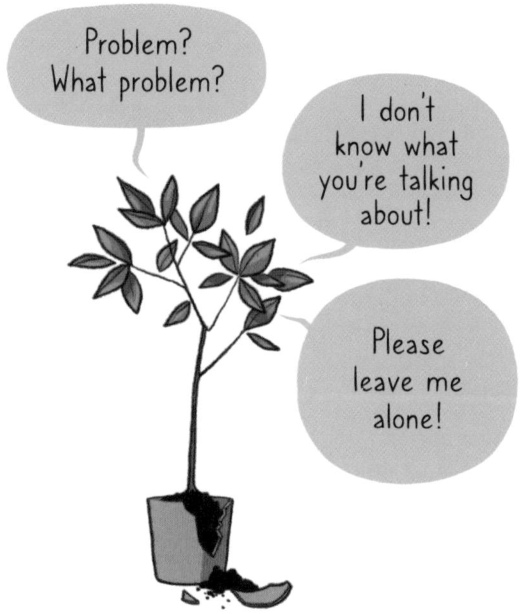
Problem? What problem?
I don't know what you're talking about!
Please leave me alone!

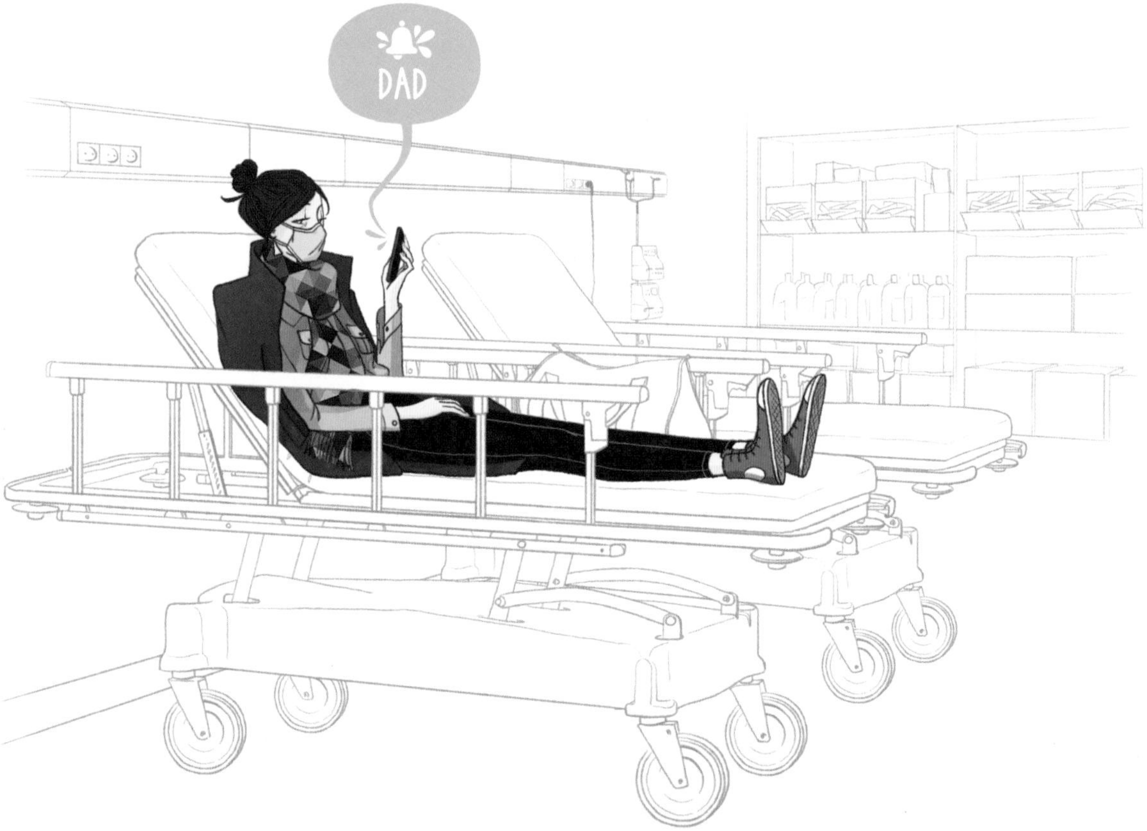
DAD

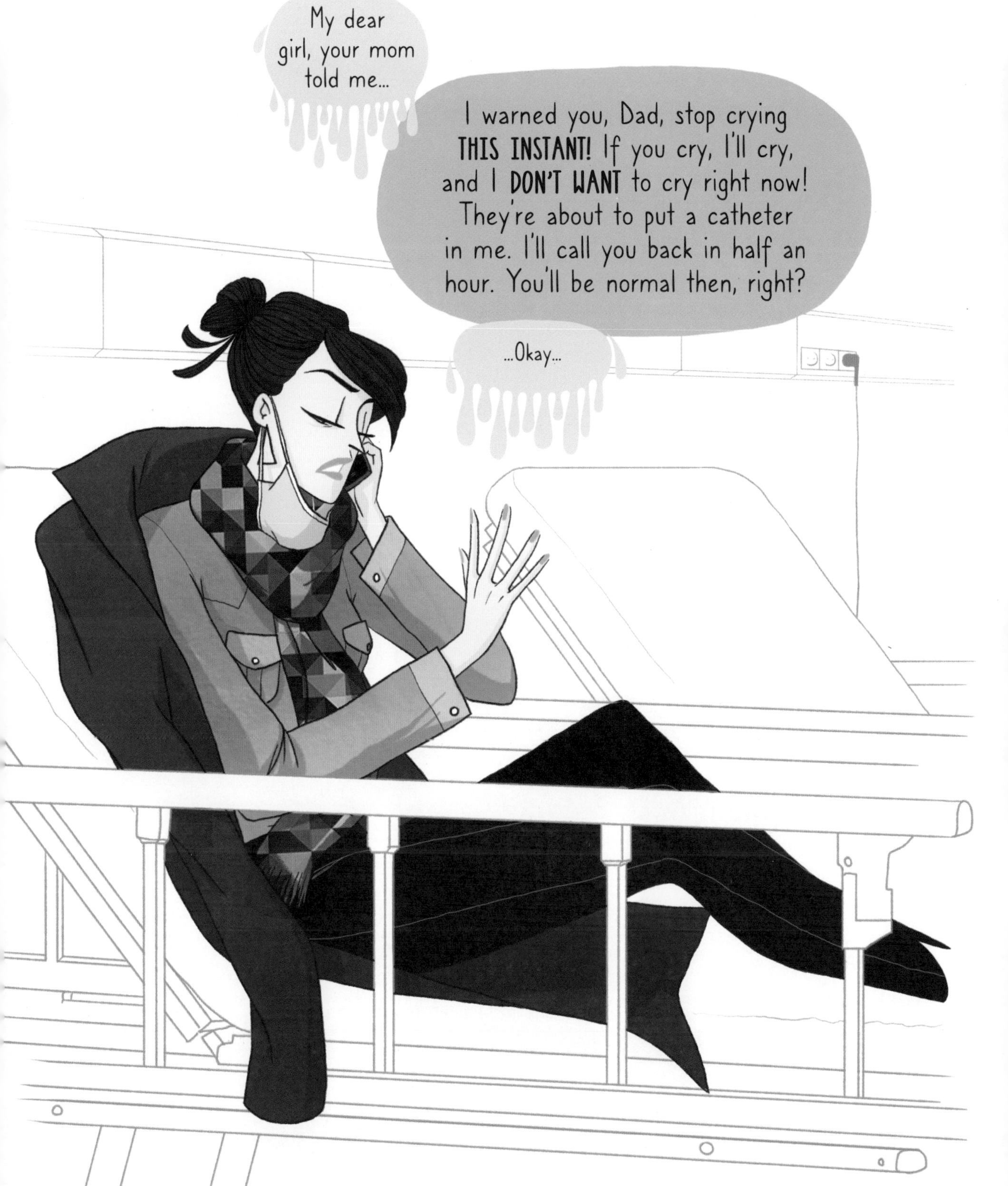

My dear girl, your mom told me...
I warned you, Dad, stop crying THIS INSTANT! If you cry, I'll cry, and I DON'T WANT to cry right now! They're about to put a catheter in me. I'll call you back in half an hour. You'll be normal then, right?
...Okay...

Chewing him out brought me back to earth and made me feel stronger and ready to face what was coming next...

WHAT CAME NEXT...

The central venous catheter is a thin, flexible tube that is inserted into a large vein near the heart. It's used to administer chemotherapy, medicines, and transfusions, and to draw blood. It's very practical and avoids pricking and damaging veins in the patient's arms (chemo products can be very toxic to veins, and there will be daily blood tests, which would do a number on the veins in the arms).

IN THEORY

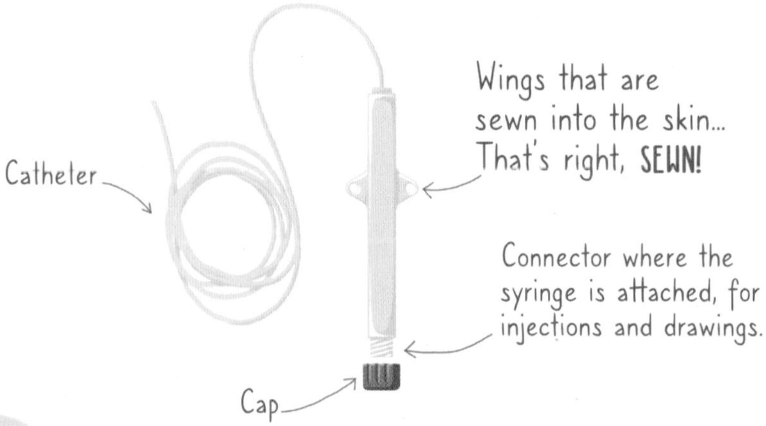
Catheter
Wings that are sewn into the skin... That's right, SEWN!
Connector where the syringe is attached, for injections and drawings.
Cap

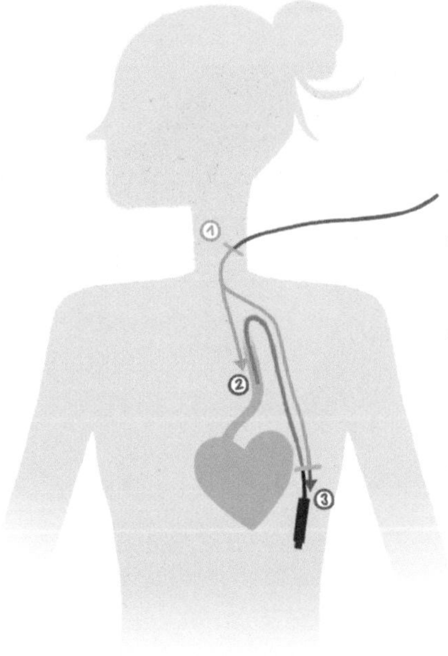

They go in through an incision in the neck.[1] One part of the catheter is then inserted into a vein going to the heart,[2] while the other part is slipped under the skin of the chest and comes back out above the breast.[3]

That's the theory, anyway. In practice, it's not quite that simple...

IN PRACTICE

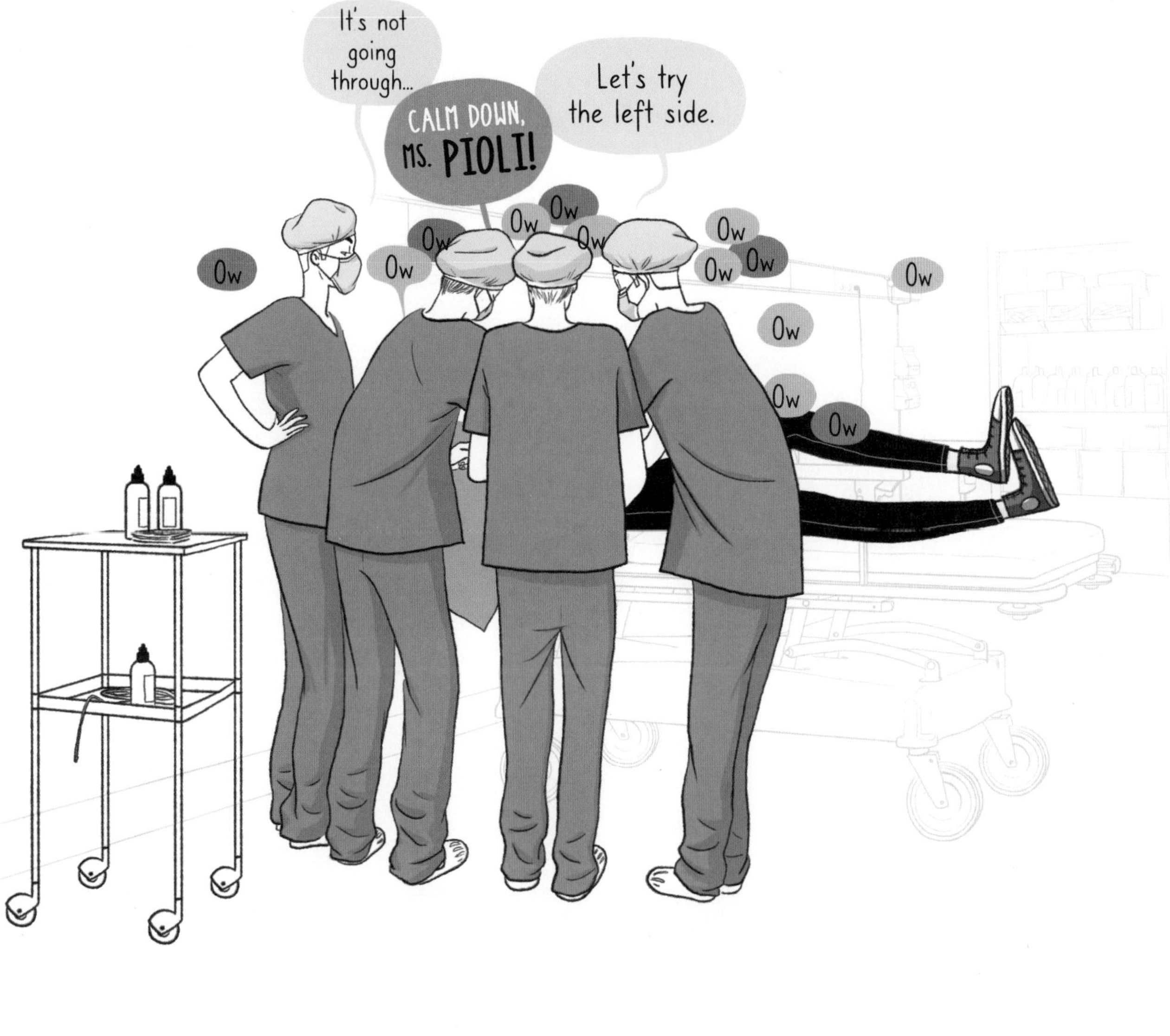

It's not going through...
CALM DOWN, MS. PIOLI!
Let's try the left side.
Ow
Ow
Ow
Ow
Ow
Ow
Ow
Ow
Ow
Ow
Ow
Ow
Ow

I'm brought to what will be my bedroom for the next 5 or 6 weeks, in the "protected" section (individual room with air filtration and positive pressure ← the filtered air circulates from my room <u>INTO</u> the hallway so no microbes come in from outside).
Visitors, including hospital personnel, are required to wear a mask.

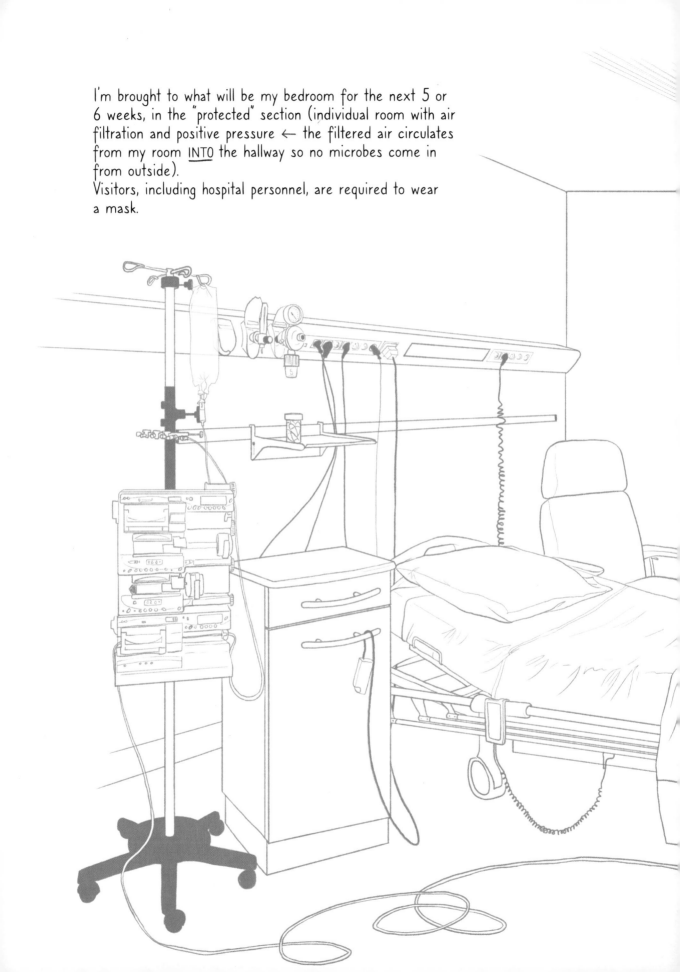

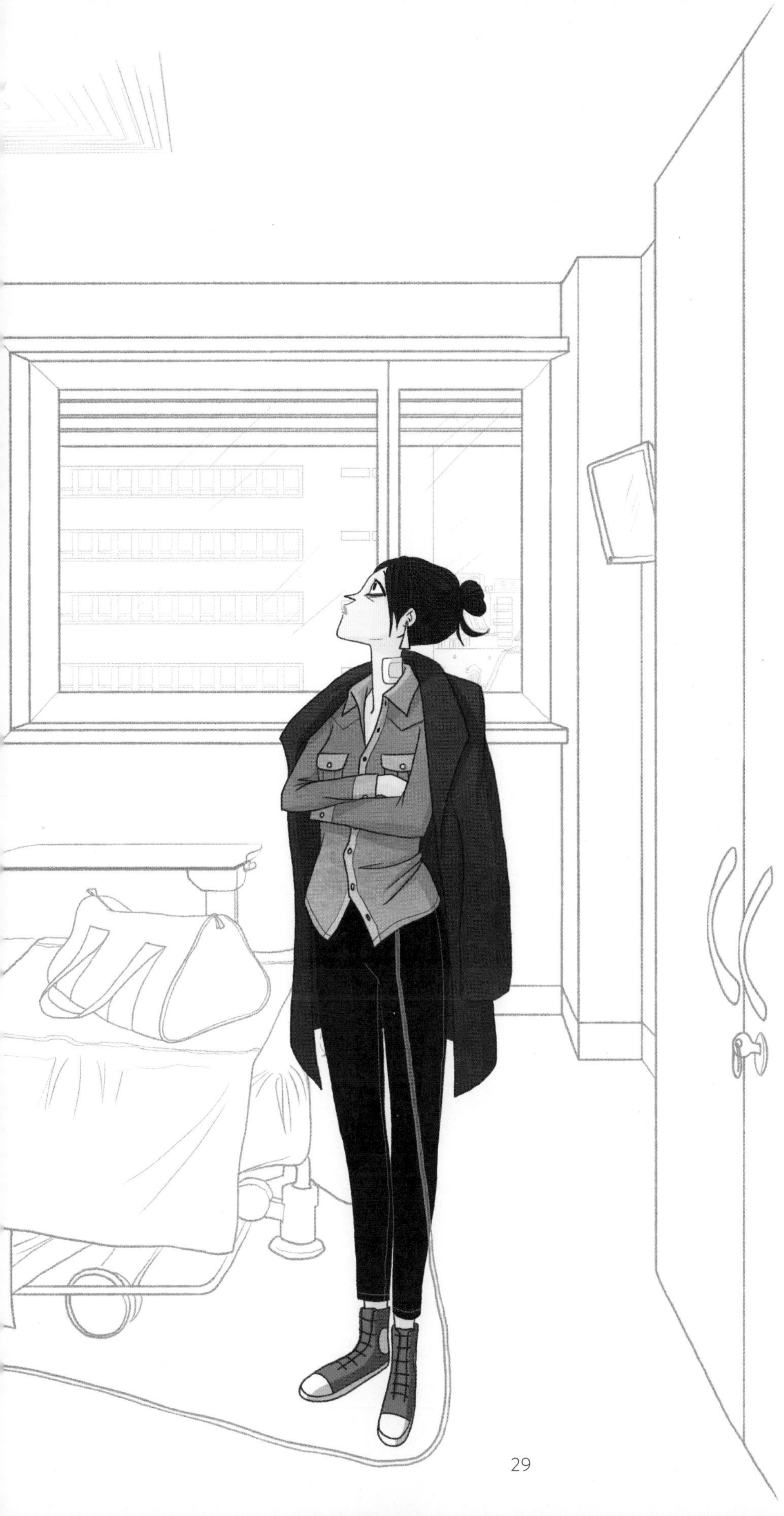

NOT CRYING...

Sébastien, my partner, can finally come see me. It does me some good but at the same time it's sad: he's the first person I **SEE** cry, and his reaction causes me to realize the gravity of my situation.

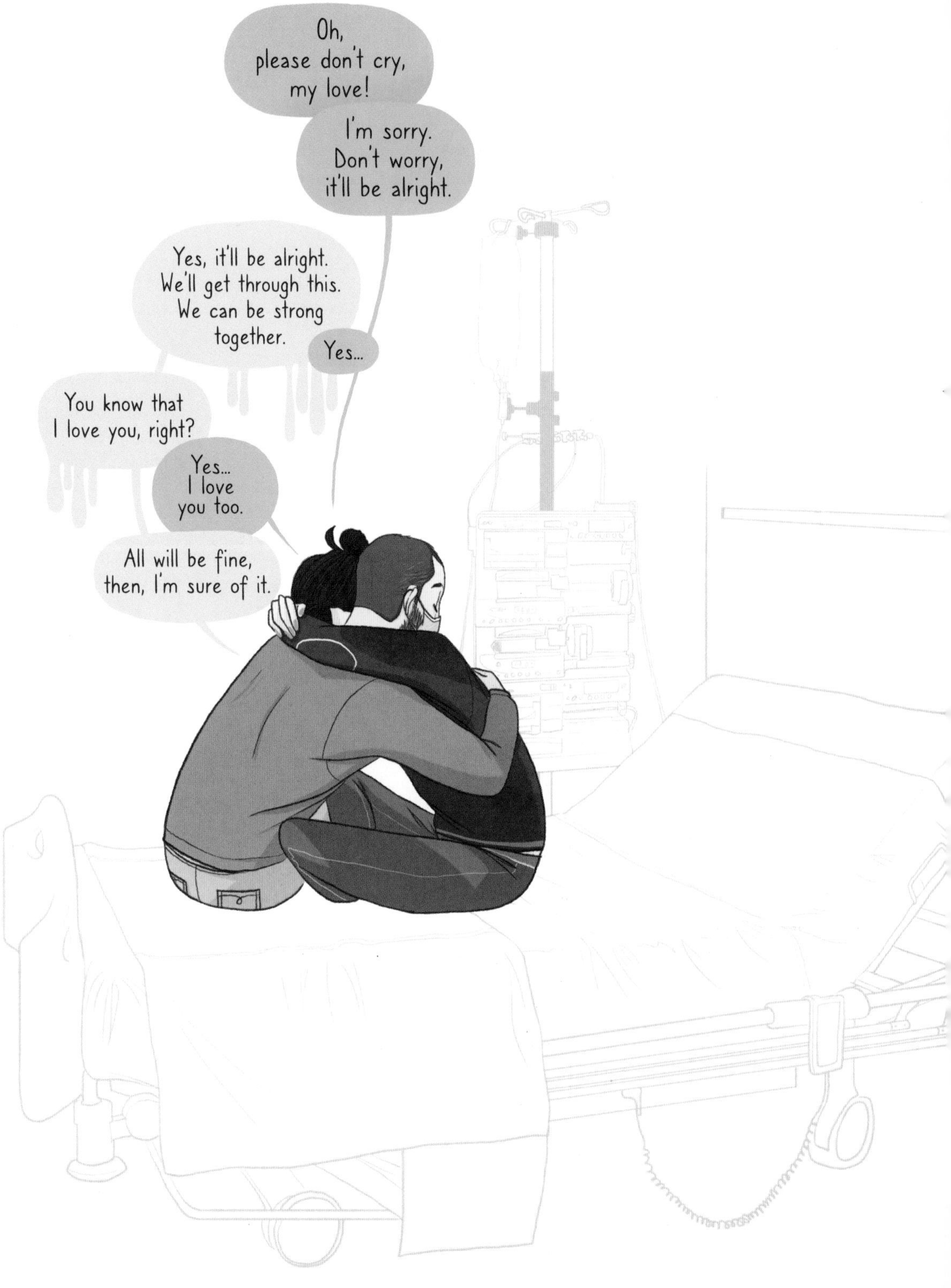

Oh, please don't cry, my love!
I'm sorry. Don't worry, it'll be alright.
Yes, it'll be alright. We'll get through this. We can be strong together.
Yes...
You know that I love you, right?
Yes... I love you too.
All will be fine, then, I'm sure of it.

...BUT LAUGHING

I'm stating the obvious, but friends are incredibly important. They play things down, laugh with you, and act like nothing's wrong.

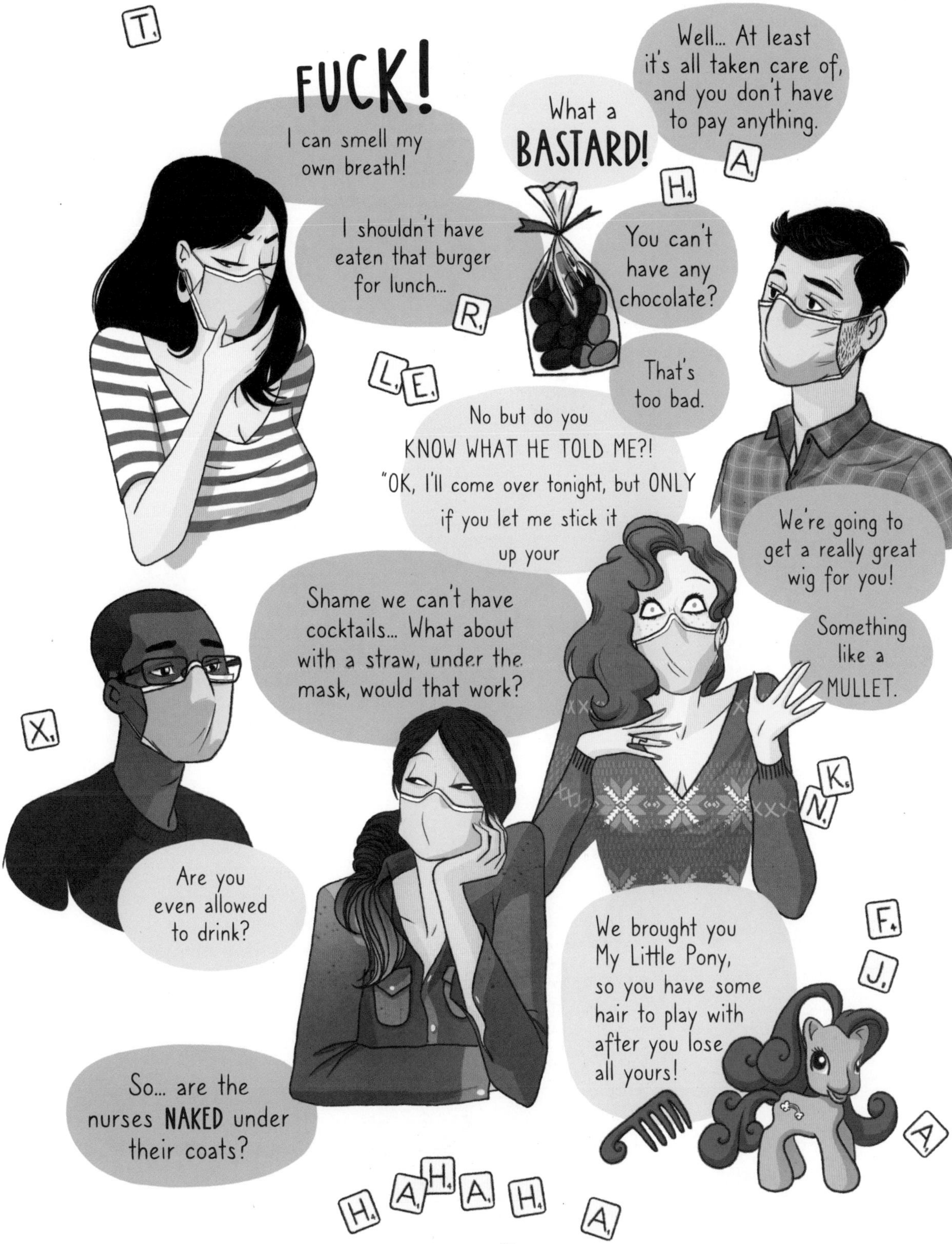
FUCK! I can smell my own breath!
I shouldn't have eaten that burger for lunch...
What a BASTARD!
Well... At least it's all taken care of, and you don't have to pay anything.
You can't have any chocolate?
That's too bad.
No but do you KNOW WHAT HE TOLD ME?! "OK, I'll come over tonight, but ONLY if you let me stick it up your
We're going to get a really great wig for you!
Something like a MULLET.
Shame we can't have cocktails... What about with a straw, under the mask, would that work?
Are you even allowed to drink?
We brought you My Little Pony, so you have some hair to play with after you lose all yours!
So... are the nurses NAKED under their coats?

THE PROBLEMS BEGIN

Before starting whatever this is, the chemo protocol (what/how much/when) has to be determined, which ends up taking almost a dozen days. During this time, my sciatica flares up. So I'm given morphine. And morphine causes constipation...

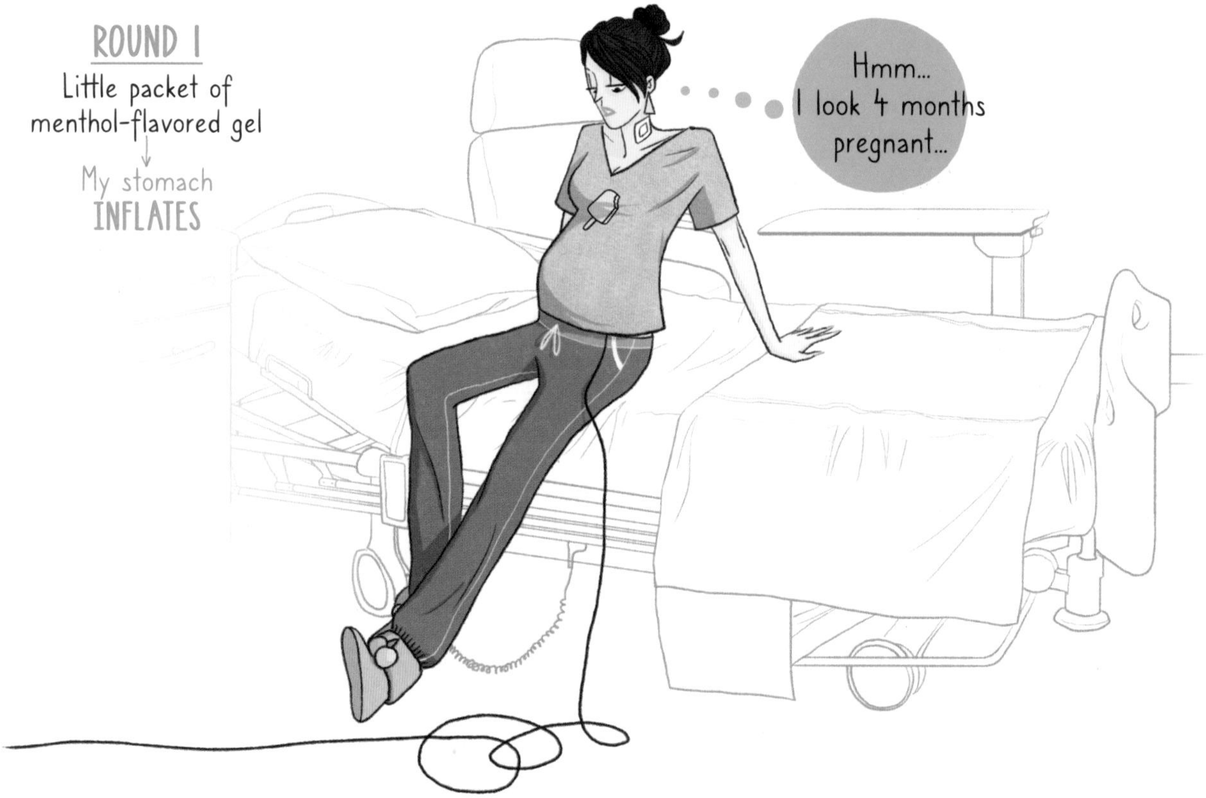
ROUND 1
Little packet of menthol-flavored gel
My stomach INFLATES
Hmm... I look 4 months pregnant...

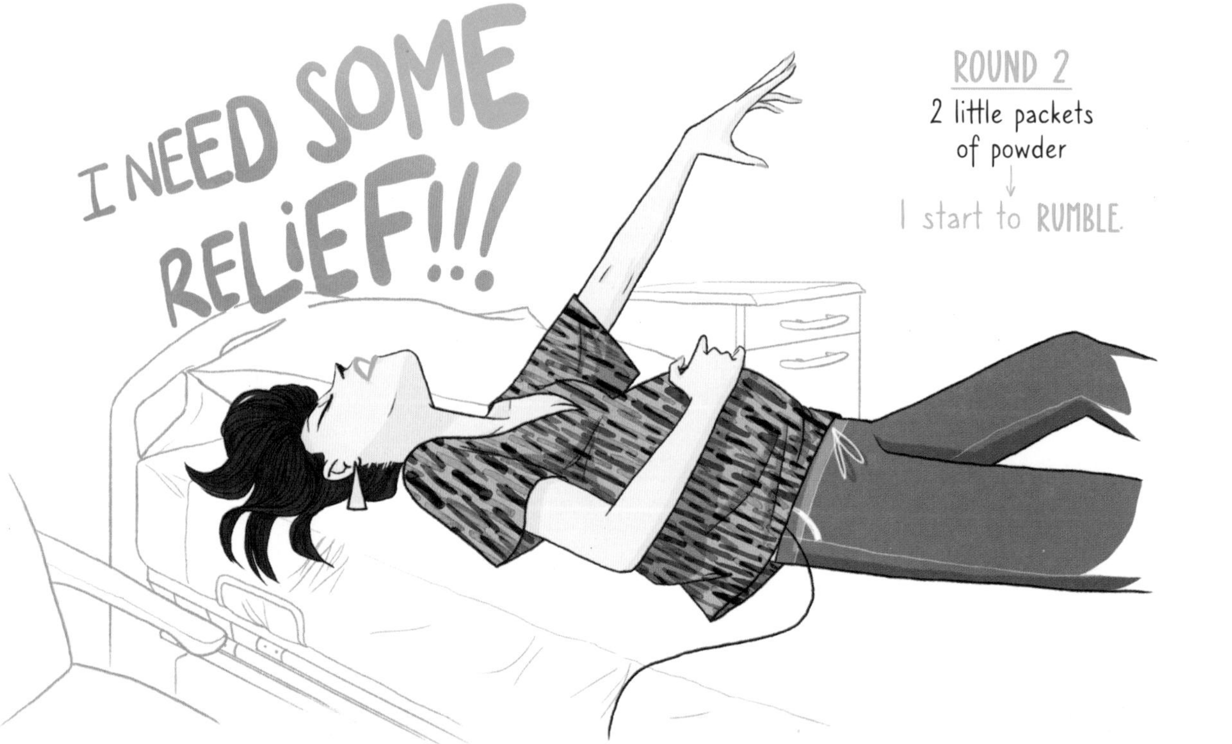
I NEED SOME RELiEF!!!
ROUND 2
2 little packets of powder
I start to RUMBLE.

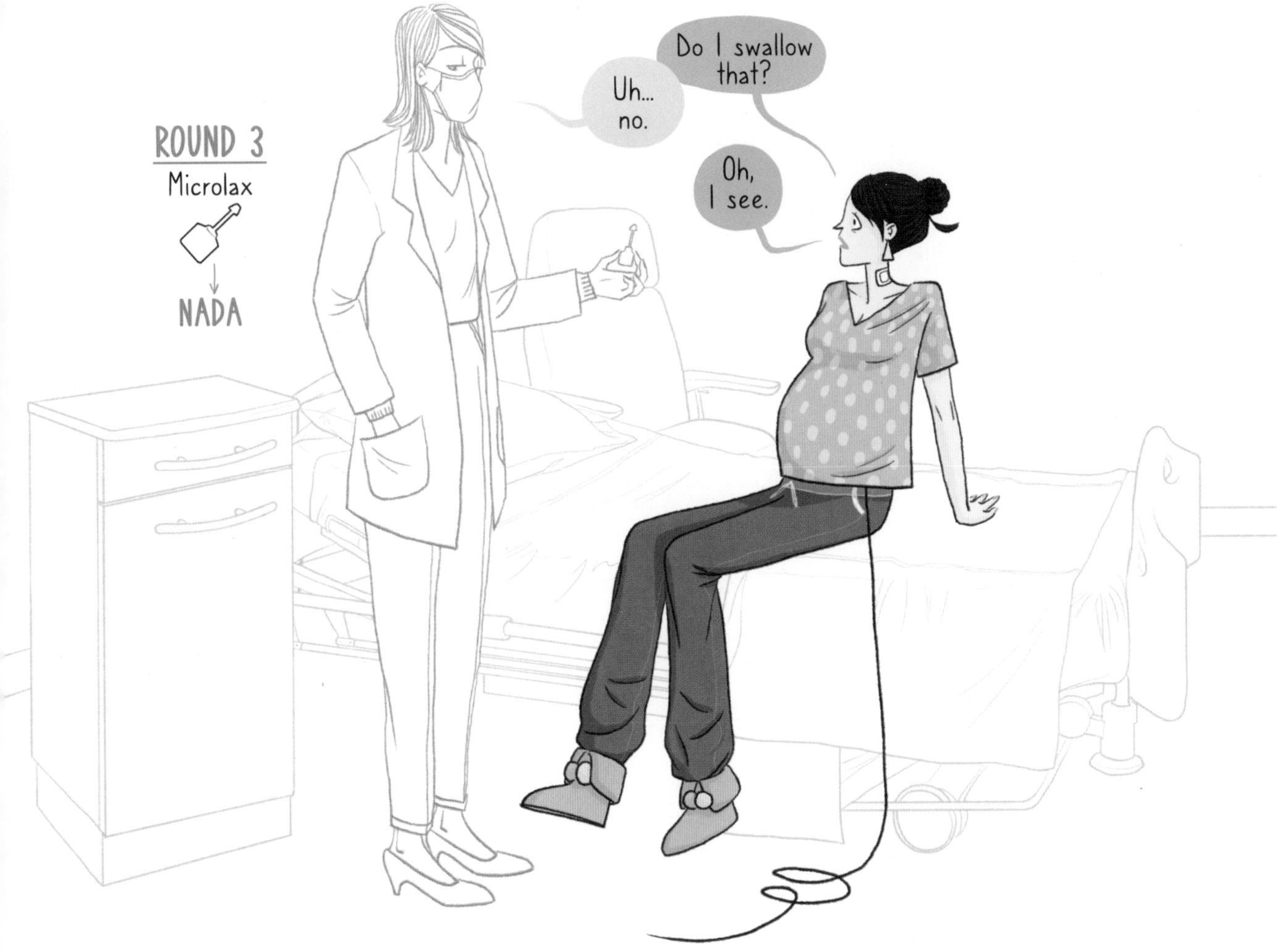
ROUND 3
Microlax
NADA
Do I swallow that?
Uh... no.
Oh, I see.

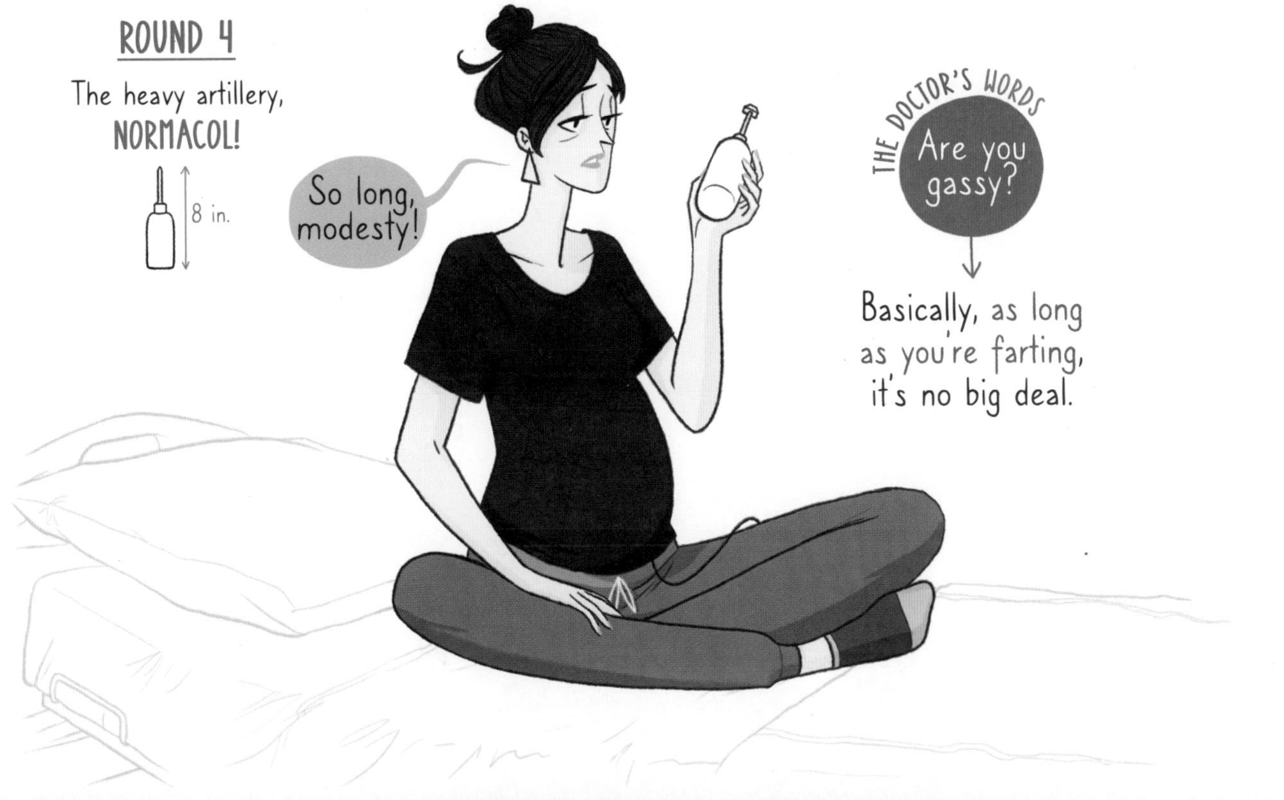
ROUND 4
The heavy artillery, NORMACOL!
8 in.
So long, modesty!
THE DOCTOR'S WORDS
Are you gassy?
Basically, as long as you're farting, it's no big deal.

THE PROBLEMS CONTINUE

To monitor my status and refine the diagnosis, there are some procedures I'll need to undergo throughout my treatment.

THE MYELOGRAM

Bone marrow is taken from the sternum and examined for contamination by cancerous cells.

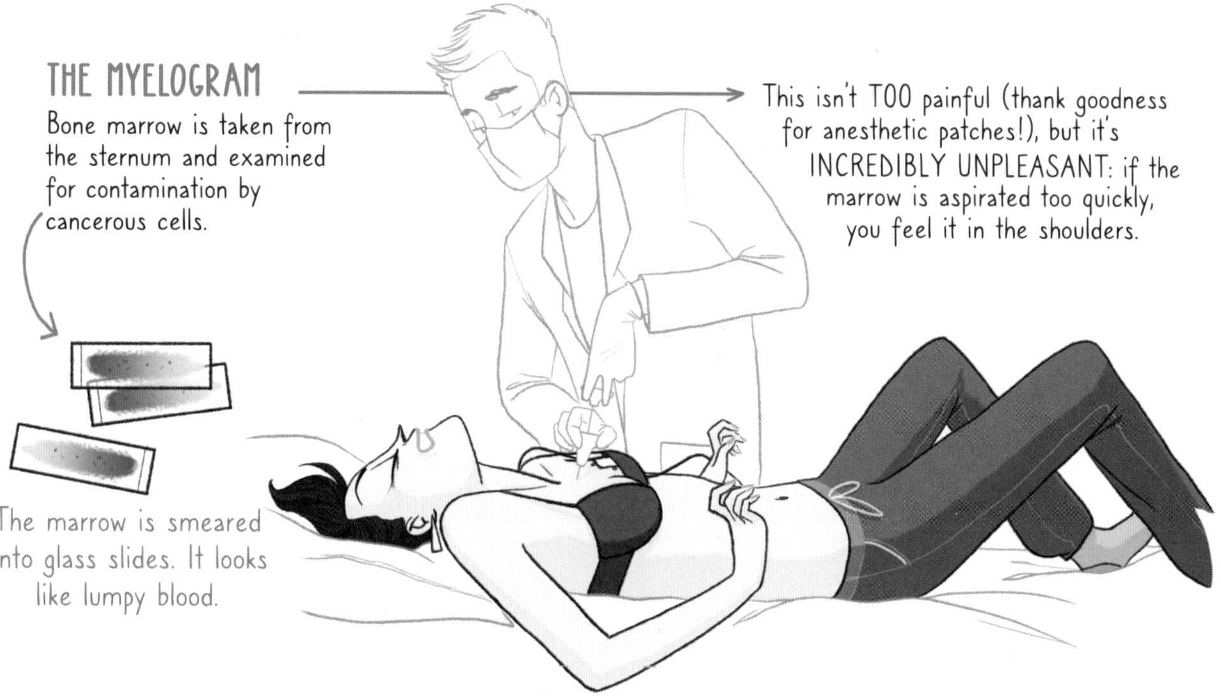
This isn't TOO painful (thank goodness for anesthetic patches!), but it's INCREDIBLY UNPLEASANT: if the marrow is aspirated too quickly, you feel it in the shoulders.
The marrow is smeared onto glass slides. It looks like lumpy blood.

THE SPINAL TAP

A syringe is inserted between two vertebrae to draw out cerebrospinal fluid and see if it has any cancerous cells.

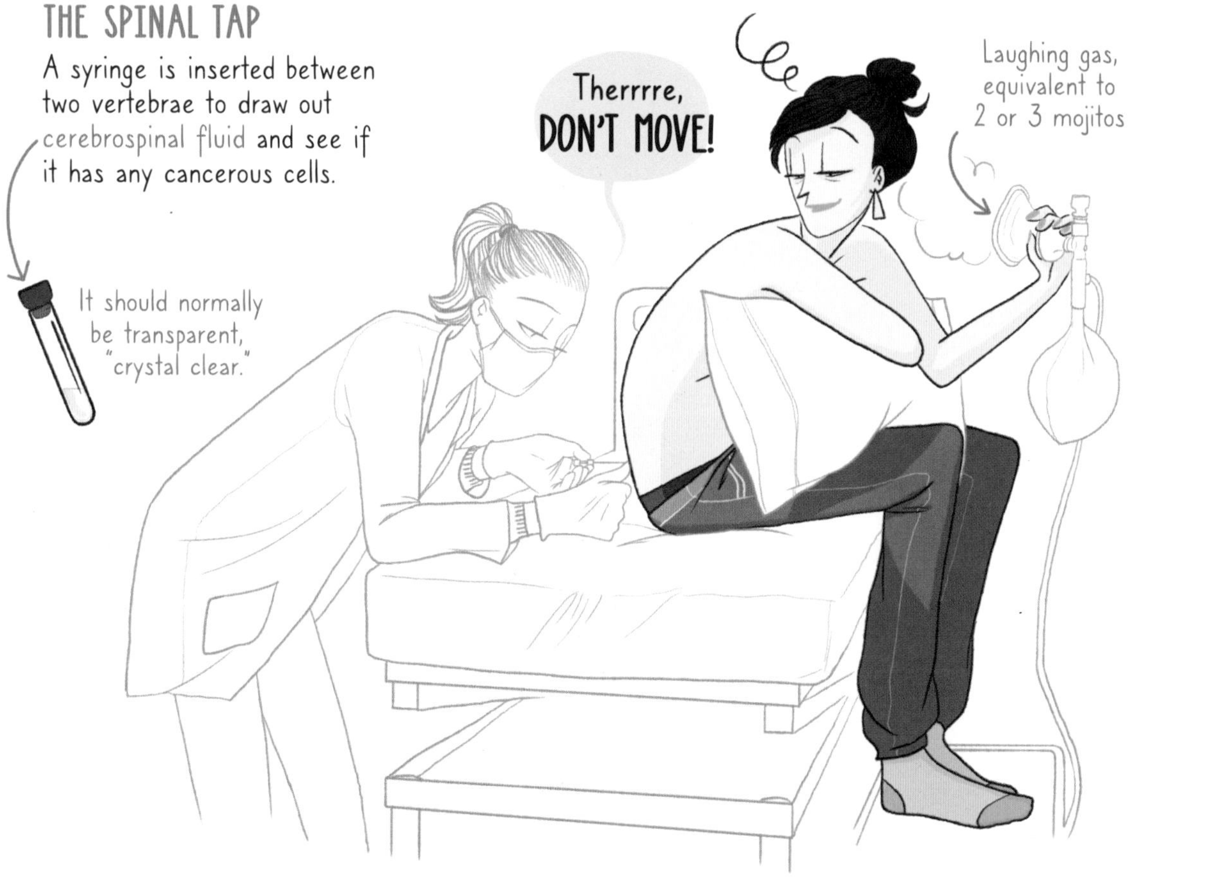
It should normally be transparent, "crystal clear."
Therrrre, DON'T MOVE!
Laughing gas, equivalent to 2 or 3 mojitos

And there you have it, my leukemia has been analyzed down to the bone (ha ha...) and identified: it turns out to be

ACUTE LYMPHOCYTIC LEUKEMIA aka ALL

with **PHILADELPHIA CHROMOSOME** (a little "East Coast" touch). The chemo protocol can now be determined. We're going to start with a big dose, to weaken the illness as much as possible... and me too, for that matter! This is called...

The iNDUCTiON Phase
ELL

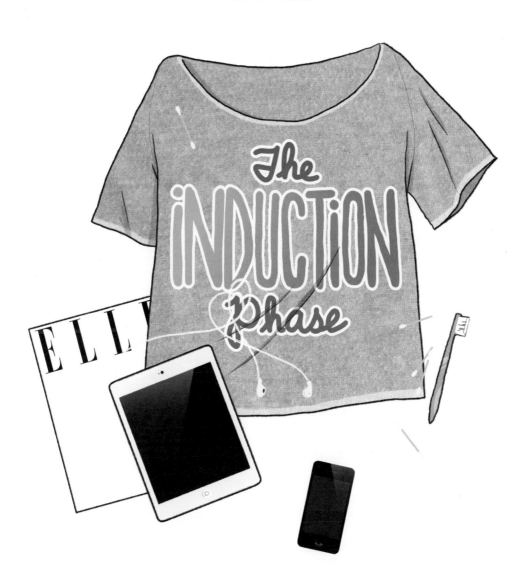

WINTER

Paris

Let's go!
HOPITAL S^T ANTOINE
LIBERTE EGALITE FRATERNITE

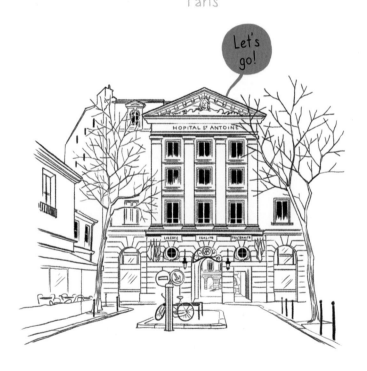

CARROT SOUP

We're finally starting chemo! I'm relieved that the eradication of my rotten cells has **TRULY** begun. The preceding phase for diagnosis and analysis was necessary but also very frustrating.

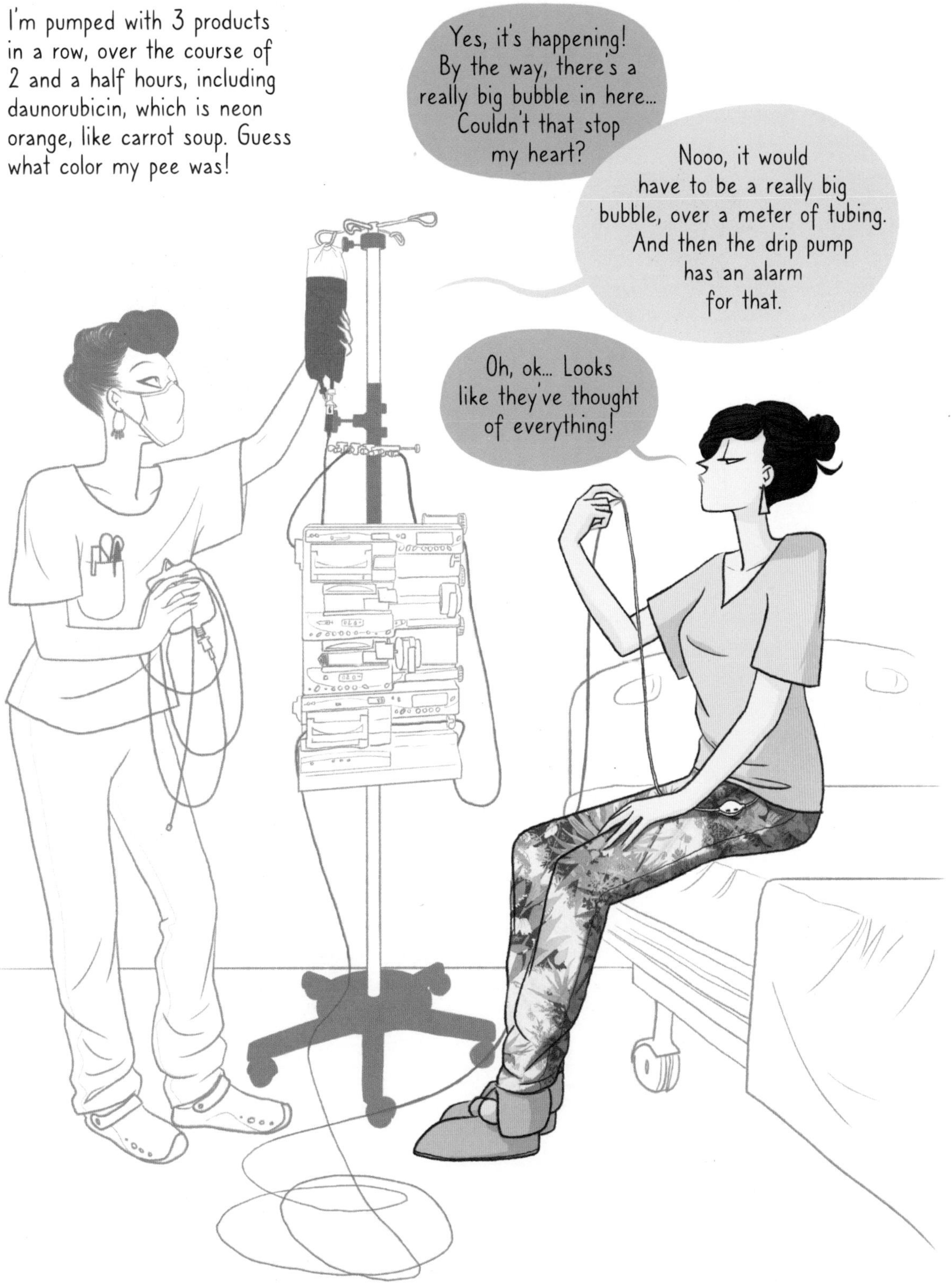

I'm pumped with 3 products in a row, over the course of 2 and a half hours, including daunorubicin, which is neon orange, like carrot soup. Guess what color my pee was!
Yes, it's happening! By the way, there's a really big bubble in here... Couldn't that stop my heart?
Nooo, it would have to be a really big bubble, over a meter of tubing. And then the drip pump has an alarm for that.
Oh, ok... Looks like they've thought of everything!

FROM BAD TO WORSE

The chemo lasts 14 days: in short, I take one kind of medicine every other day, and once a week, all the medicines together. I'm a little "disappointed," since the entire process seems short to me and I might still have diseased cells. I've been at the hospital for nearly a month and it's starting to weigh on me.

The routine becomes... unbearable.

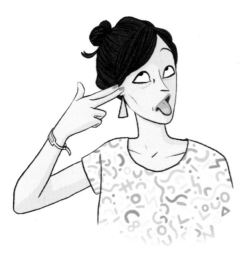

I've lost all appetite.
I'm only given bananas and cottage cheese.
Smells disgust me.

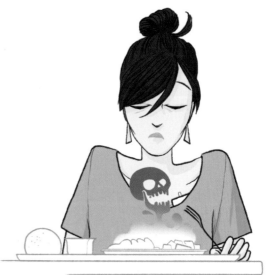

Swallowing anything is a chore. Taking my medications or even using mouthwash makes me want to vomit.

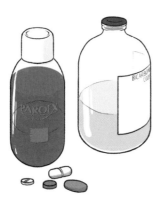

The nausea is constant.
And throwing up banana is frankly revolting...

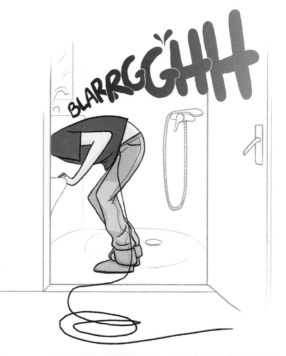

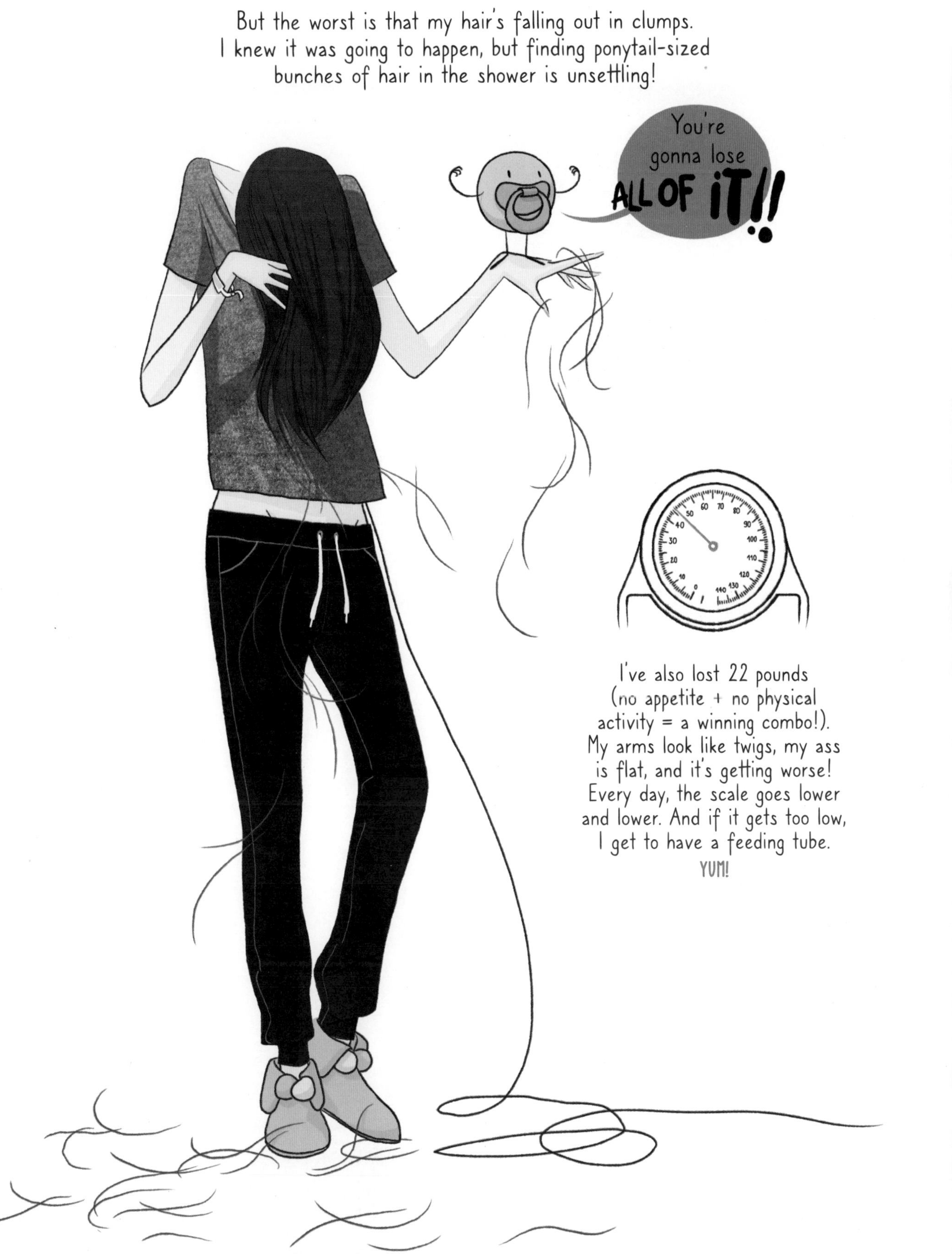
But the worst is that my hair's falling out in clumps. I knew it was going to happen, but finding ponytail-sized bunches of hair in the shower is unsettling!
You're gonna lose ALL OF IT!!
I've also lost 22 pounds (no appetite + no physical activity = a winning combo!). My arms look like twigs, my ass is flat, and it's getting worse! Every day, the scale goes lower and lower. And if it gets too low, I get to have a feeding tube.
YUM!

GROWN-UP CHILDREN, GROWN-UP PROBLEMS

My parents both live in Corsica, so they haven't been able to come see me right away.
I think this must have worried them even more.

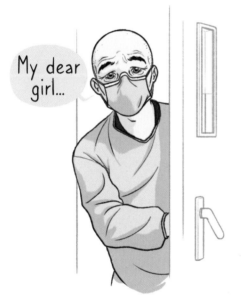

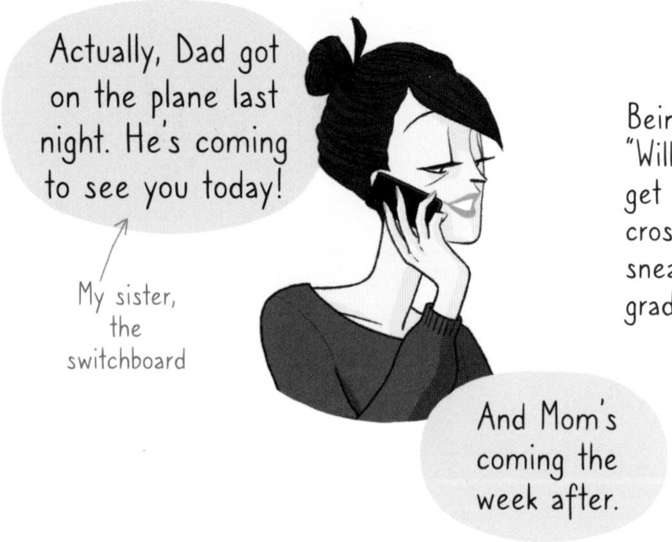

Actually, Dad got on the plane last night. He's coming to see you today!

My sister, the switchboard

And Mom's coming the week after.

Being a parent means worrying.
"Will my child sleep through the night/get into day care/look both ways before crossing/make friends at school/smoke/sneak booze/get hooked on drugs/get good grades/find a job...?" The list goes on.

My dear girl...

As adults, we forget that our parents worry about us, even if it's still the case.

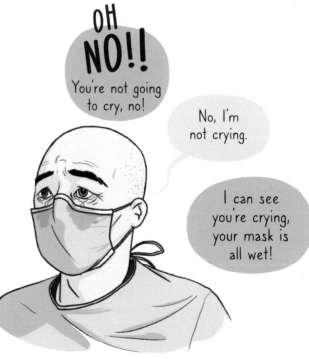

OH NO!! You're not going to cry, no!

No, I'm not crying.

I can see you're crying, your mask is all wet!

We have a career, we don't live with them anymore, we live separate lives from them, at least physically. So we stop thinking about their worrying.

And so we forget.

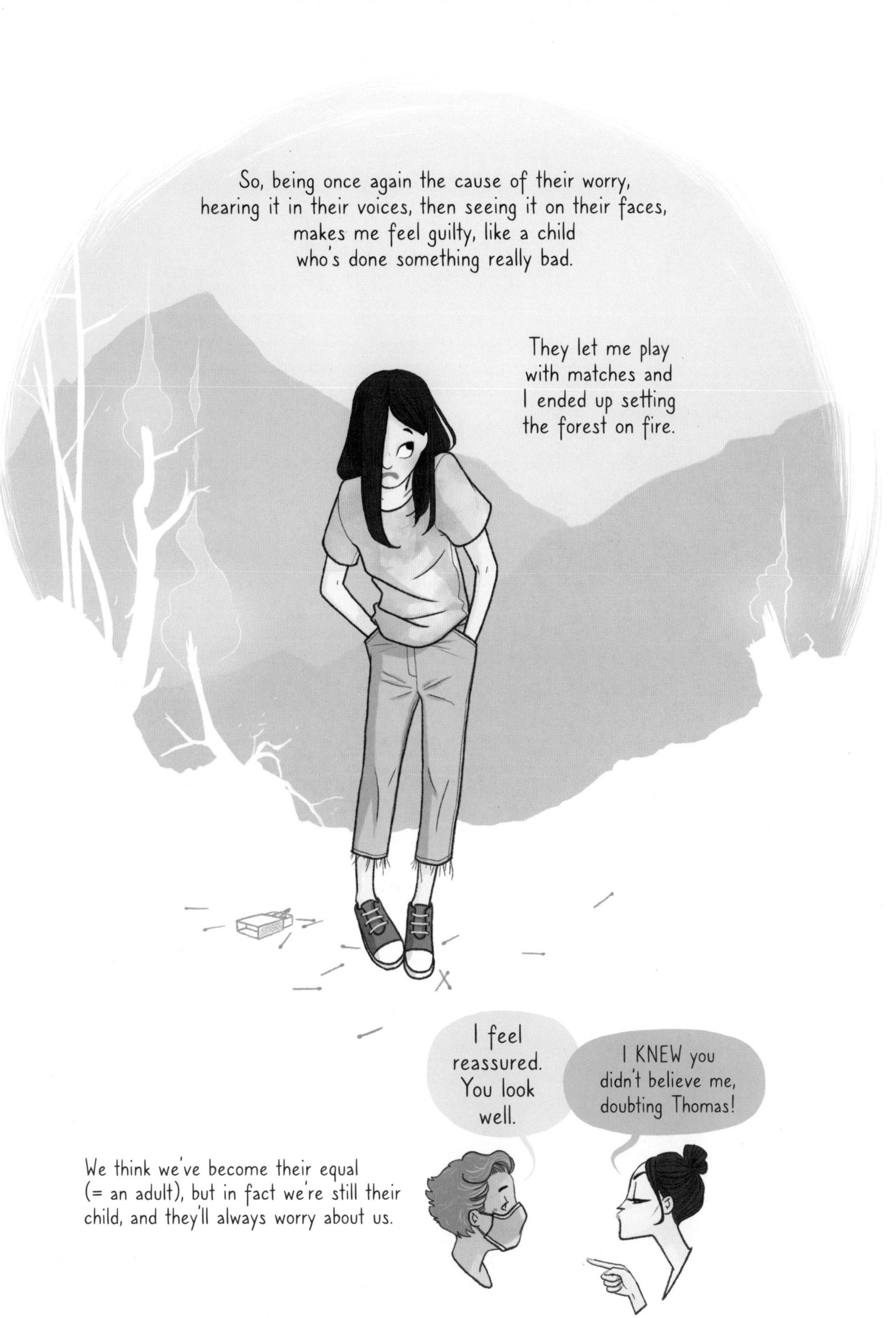
So, being once again the cause of their worry, hearing it in their voices, then seeing it on their faces, makes me feel guilty, like a child who's done something really bad.
They let me play with matches and I ended up setting the forest on fire.
I feel reassured. You look well.
I KNEW you didn't believe me, doubting Thomas!
We think we've become their equal (= an adult), but in fact we're still their child, and they'll always worry about us.

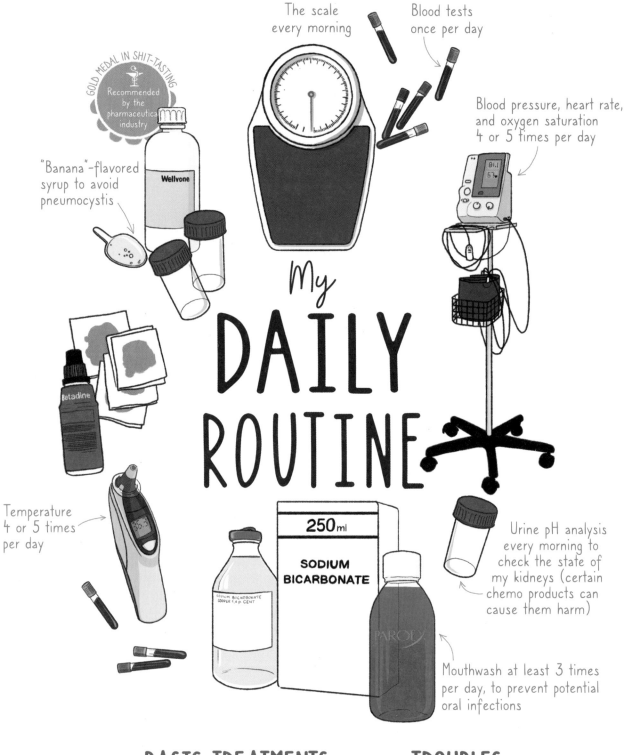

The scale every morning

Blood tests once per day

GOLD MEDAL IN SHIT-TASTING
Recommended by the pharmaceutical industry

Blood pressure, heart rate, and oxygen saturation 4 or 5 times per day

"Banana"-flavored syrup to avoid pneumocystis

Wellvone

My DAILY ROUTINE

Betadine

Temperature 4 or 5 times per day

250 ml

SODIUM BICARBONATE

SODIUM BICARBONATE COOPER 1.4 p CENT

PAROL

Urine pH analysis every morning to check the state of my kidneys (certain chemo products can cause them harm)

Mouthwash at least 3 times per day, to prevent potential oral infections

BASIC TREATMENTS TO AVOID ANY NUMBER OF TROUBLES

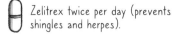 Zelitrex twice per day (prevents shingles and herpes).

 Luteran, to stop menstruation (because of my low platelet count, there's a risk of hemorrhage).

Glivec, anticancer medicine.

Inexium, to protect the stomach.

Loramyc, for fungal mouth infections, applied to the gums before going to bed.

Fortunately, all the nurses are really nice. I was expecting to be treated like a child ("How's our young lady today?"), but no! They're kind, attentive, and take an interest in me beyond my illness. I only see them from behind their masks, and I wonder if the way I imagine their faces conforms to reality. I'm lost in a sea of blue smocks and masked, friendly, attentive faces.

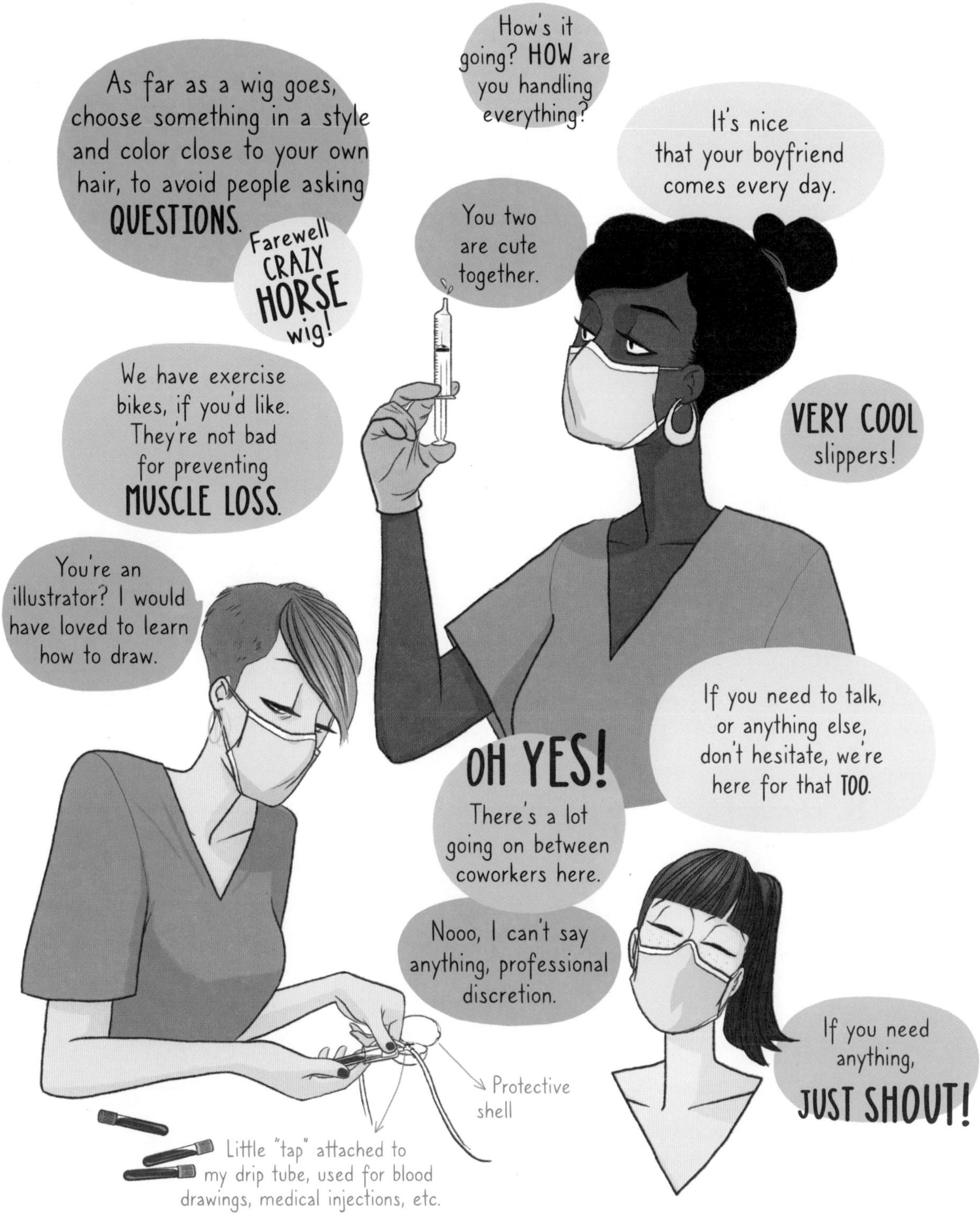

As far as a wig goes, choose something in a style and color close to your own hair, to avoid people asking QUESTIONS.
Farewell CRAZY HORSE wig!
How's it going? HOW are you handling everything?
It's nice that your boyfriend comes every day.
You two are cute together.
We have exercise bikes, if you'd like. They're not bad for preventing MUSCLE LOSS.
VERY COOL slippers!
You're an illustrator? I would have loved to learn how to draw.
If you need to talk, or anything else, don't hesitate, we're here for that TOO.
OH YES! There's a lot going on between coworkers here.
Nooo, I can't say anything, professional discretion.
If you need anything, JUST SHOUT!
Protective shell
Little "tap" attached to my drip tube, used for blood drawings, medical injections, etc.

THE ROUTINE

I'm not allowed to leave the room, and boredom has set in very quickly.
Every day feels the same, despite visits from friends and family. I struggle
to get used to this new environment. Too much to digest. Feels
like I've fallen down Alice's rabbit hole to Wonderland.

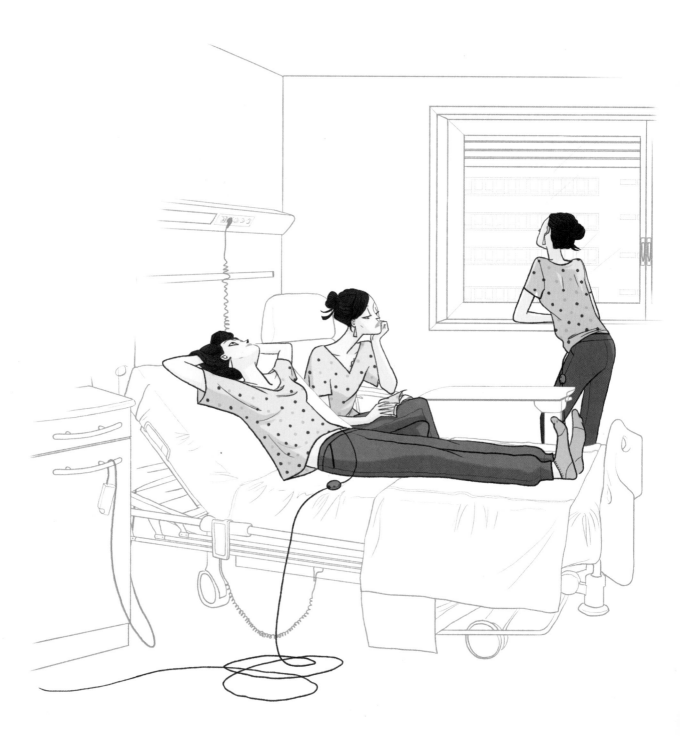

Evening is my favorite time of day. The night nurse comes by at 10 for the last blood pressure/temperature check and draws some blood (to have results ready in the morning). Then, unless there's a problem, I'm left alone until the next morning, at 6. No more visits, tests, tubes to change, beeping machines, medications, mouthwash... I'm finally ALONE! Sometimes, I leave the blinds open to watch the lights in the other hospital buildings. I see patients in their rooms, nurses, and the blue glow of televisions.

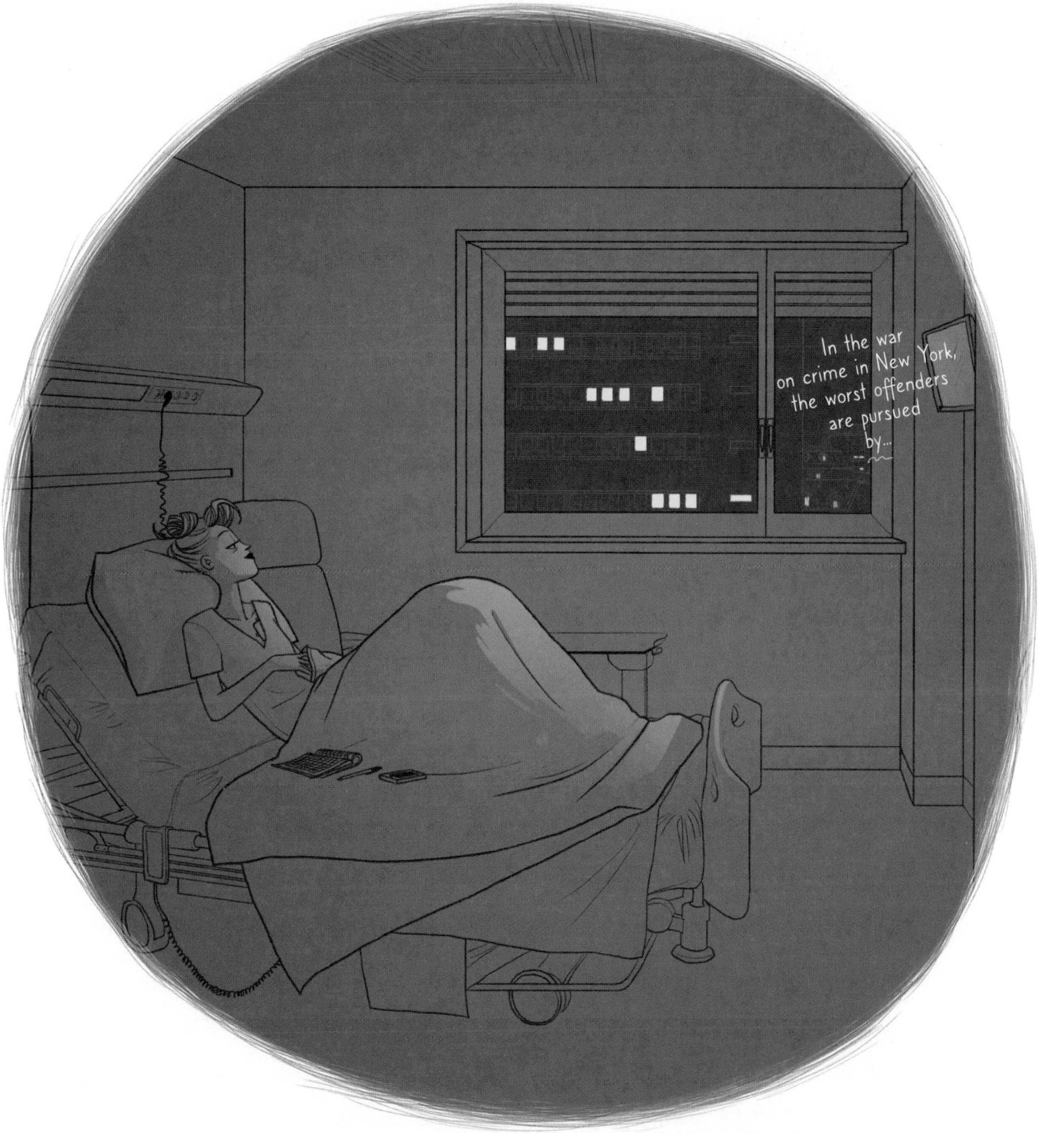
In the war on crime in New York, the worst offenders are pursued by...

COLONIZED

I ask questions—not only of the nurses, but also of the doctors.
I don't know about you, but for me, science class was a long time ago...

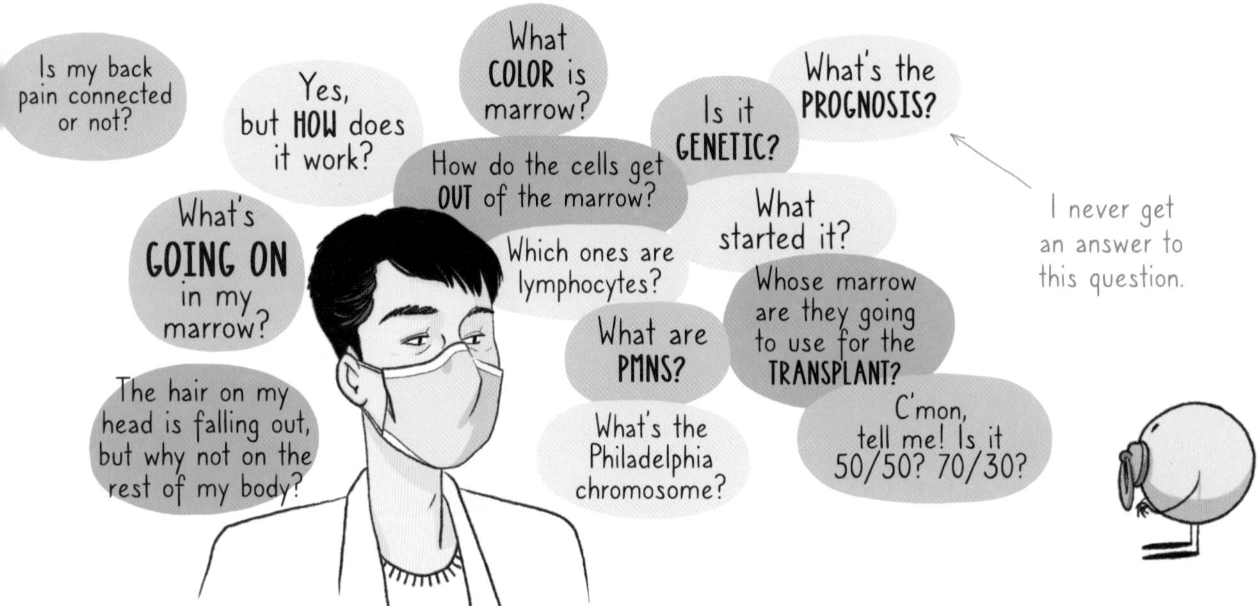

Is my back pain connected or not?
Yes, but HOW does it work?
What COLOR is marrow?
What's the PROGNOSIS?
Is it GENETIC?
How do the cells get OUT of the marrow?
What started it?
What's GOING ON in my marrow?
Which ones are lymphocytes?
Whose marrow are they going to use for the TRANSPLANT?
What are PMNS?
The hair on my head is falling out, but why not on the rest of my body?
What's the Philadelphia chromosome?
C'mon, tell me! Is it 50/50? 70/30?
I never get an answer to this question.

TO SIMPLIFY, bone marrow produces

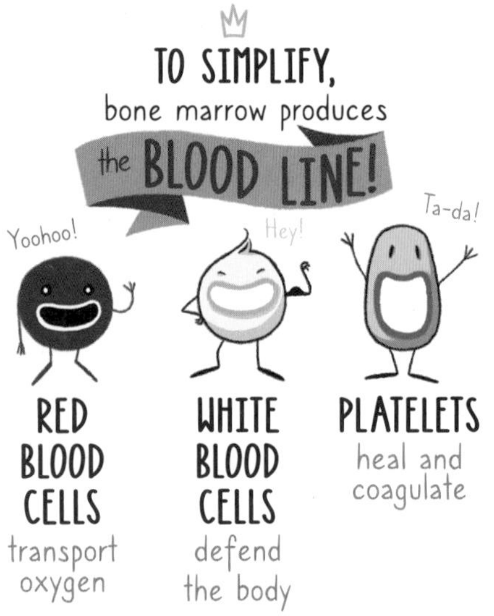

the BLOOD LINE!
Yoohoo!
Hey!
Ta-da!
RED BLOOD CELLS
transport oxygen
WHITE BLOOD CELLS
defend the body
PLATELETS
heal and coagulate

But before becoming corpuscles, these cells are **STEM CELLS,** which is to say undifferentiated, immature blood cells.

In the case of leukemia, the marrow doesn't work right and produces too many stem cells or "diseased" cells called **BLASTS.** They remain in this immature phase and take up space, doing nothing.

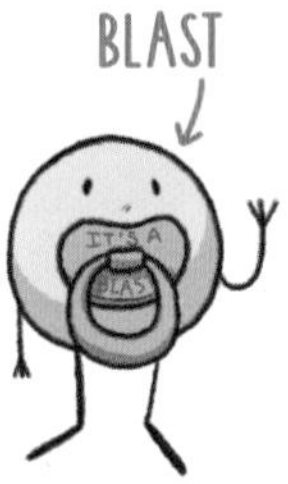

BLAST

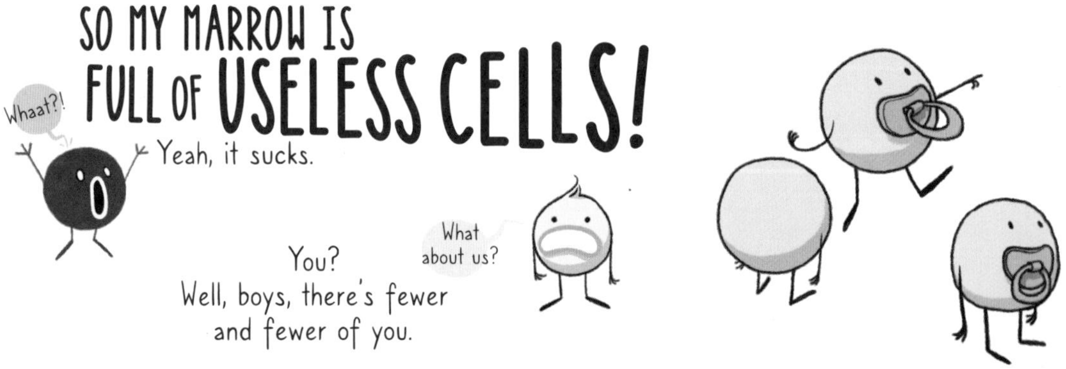

SO MY MARROW IS FULL OF USELESS CELLS!
Whaat?!
Yeah, it sucks.
What about us?
You? Well, boys, there's fewer and fewer of you.

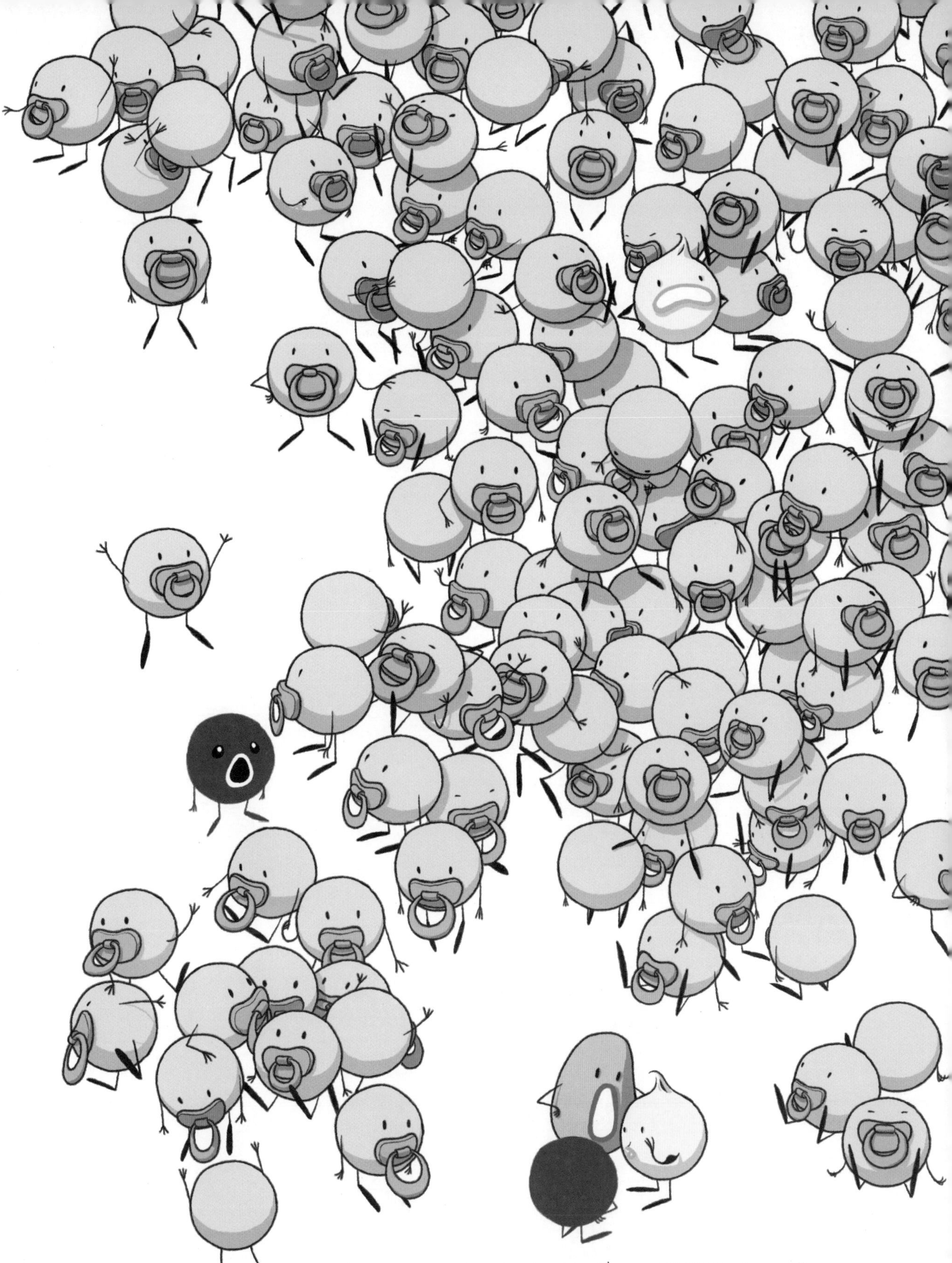

Inside me, as I understand it, it's my **LYMPHOID** stem cells (which are supposed to turn into **LYMPHOCYTES**, a type of white blood cell) that are causing the problem.

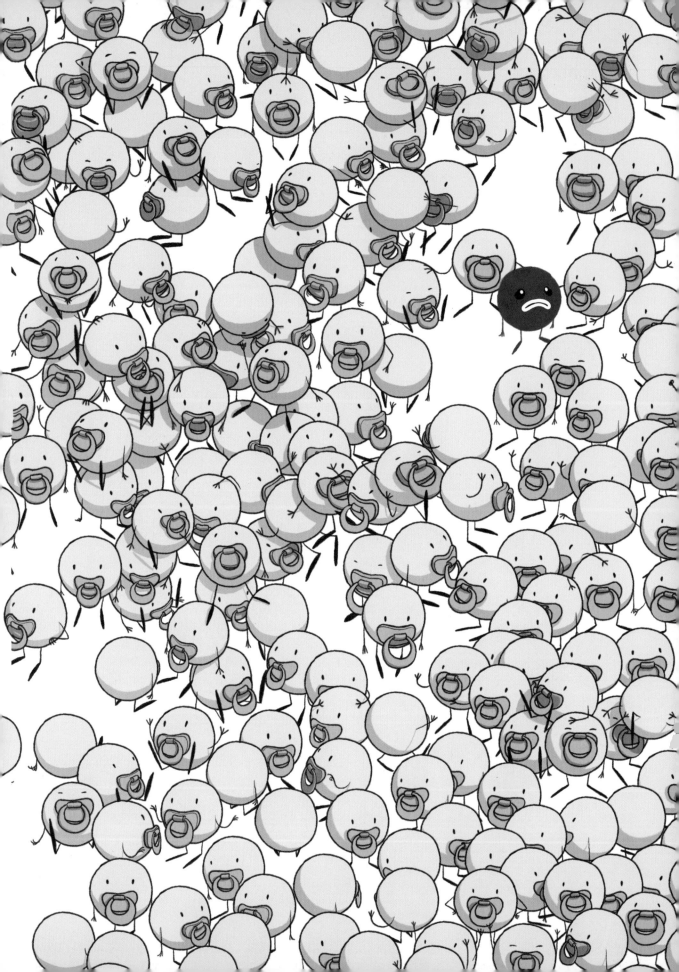

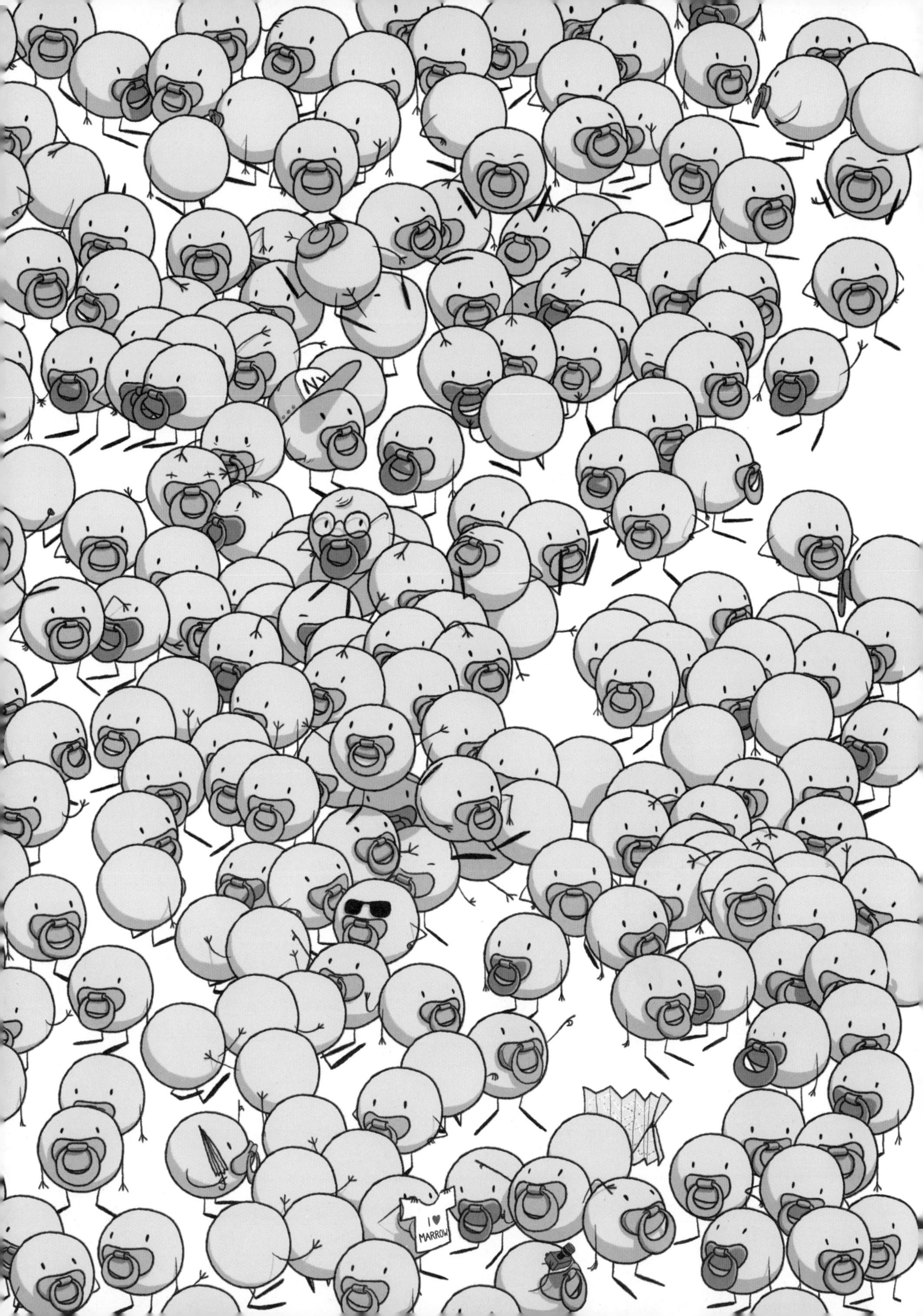
NY
I ♥ MARROW

THE GREAT CIRCUS

I can really feel the fragility of my body through all these "side" pains: nausea, lack of appetite, fatigue, dry skin, hair falling out, isolation within the hospital, my powerlessness in the face of my own defective cells... The impregnable fortress that was my body until now is taking on water from every direction. The west wing has just been trampled by savage hordes, there are infiltrations at the foundation, and the load-bearing walls are infested with termites. Everything is crumbling...

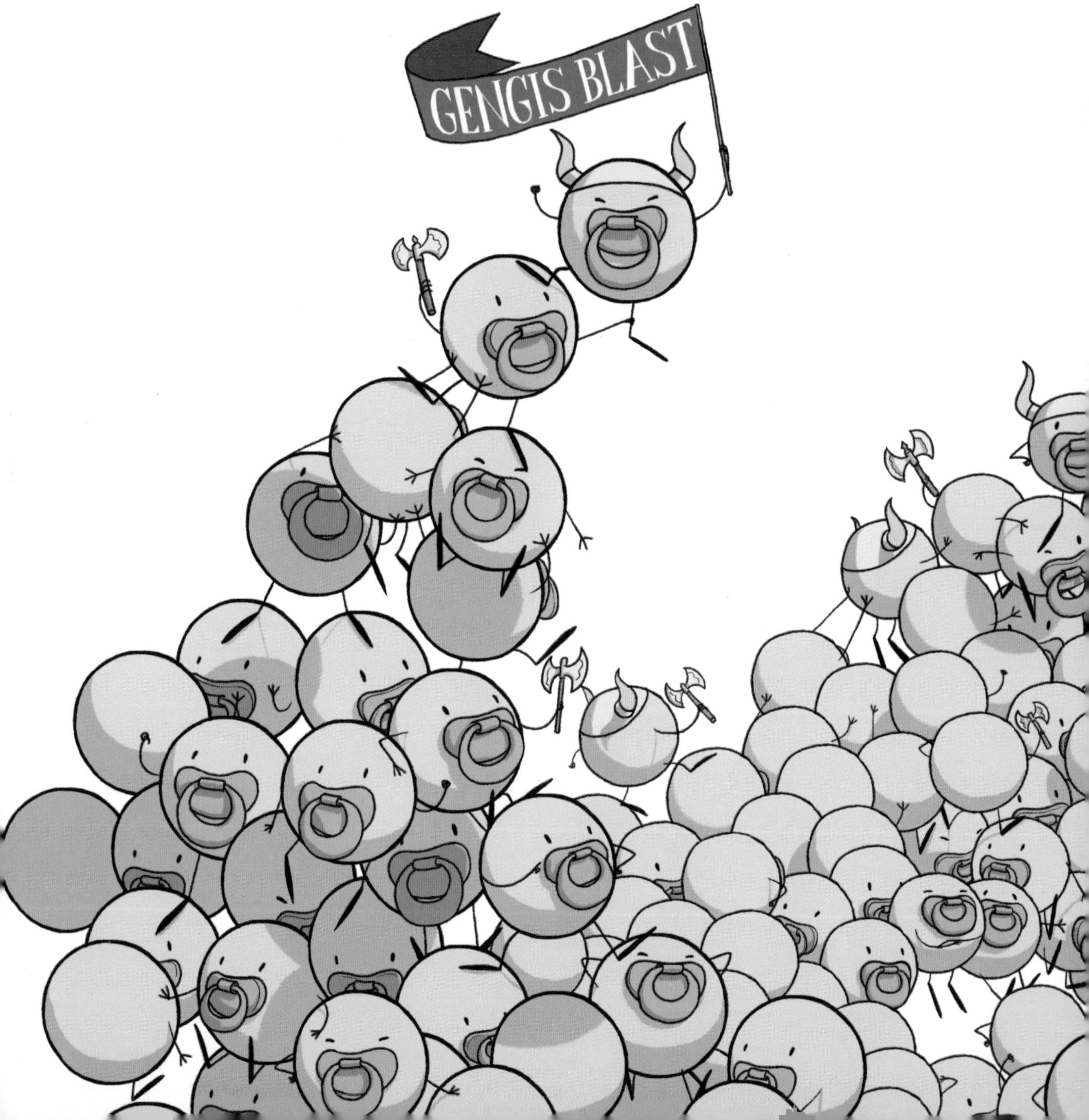
GENGIS BLAST

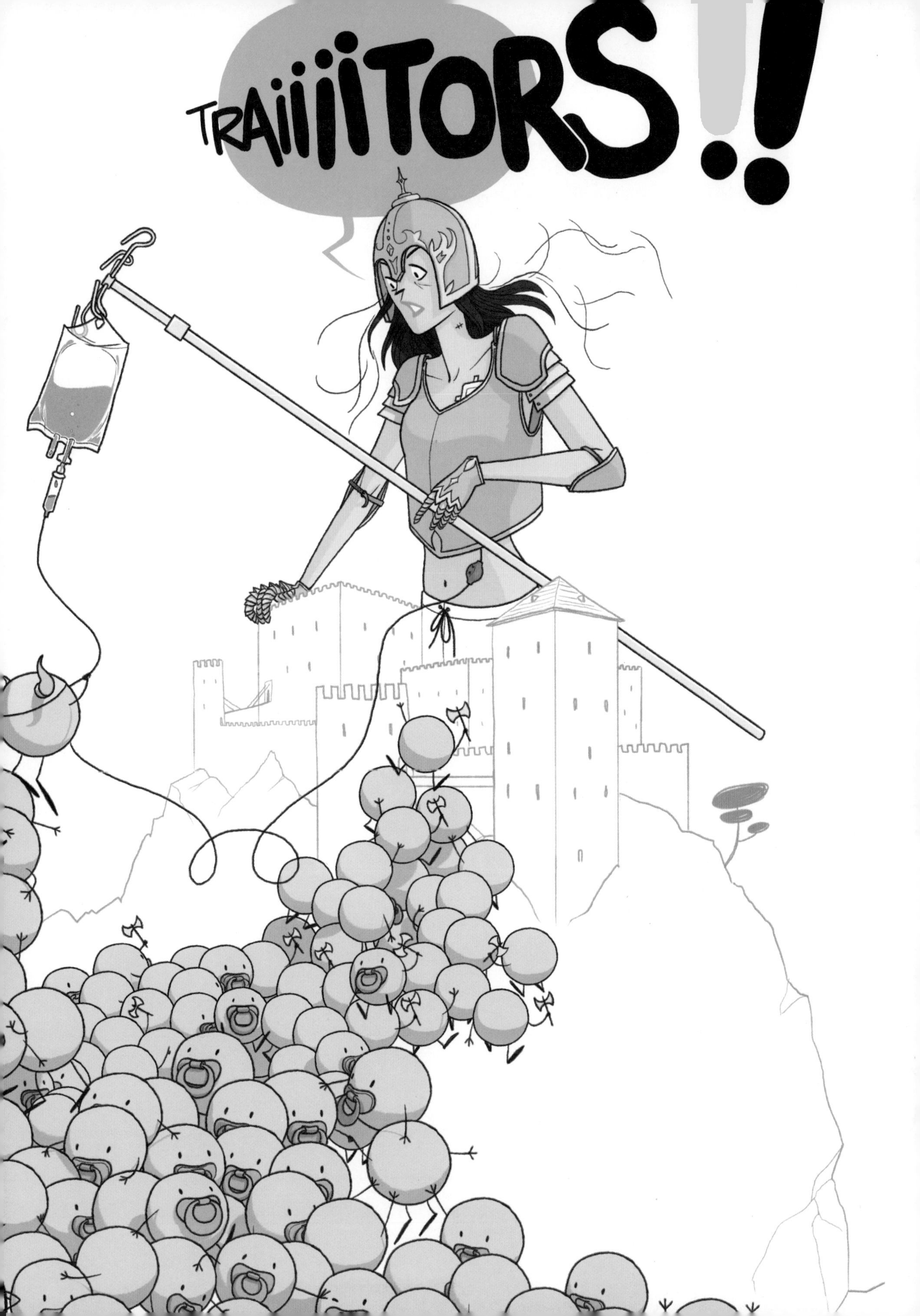
TRAiiiiiTORS!!

A BIT OF GEOGRAPHY

WHAT'S THIS PHILADELPHIA CHROMOSOME?

Well, it's a genetic exchange between chromosomes 9 and 22 in the cells of the bone marrow. The BCR and ABL genes combine and form the chimeric gene BCR-ABL. This is an aggravating factor because the new gene disrupts cellular division and makes the illness more aggressive and more likely to recur. This mutation is present in 20% to 30% of cases of ALL.

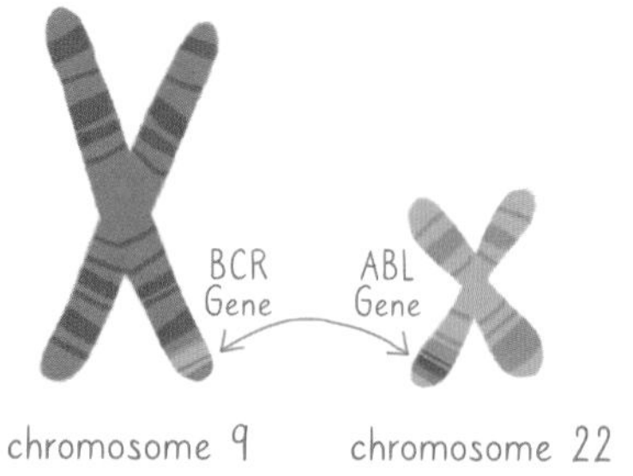
BCR Gene
ABL Gene
chromosome 9
chromosome 22

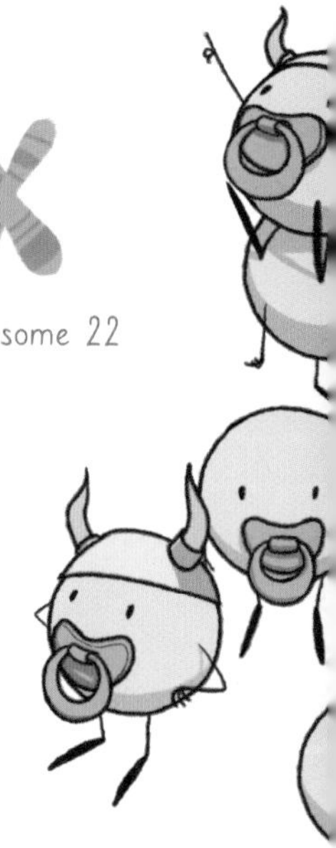

HOW DOES IT WORK?

BCR-ABL frees a type of protein, tyrosine kinase, a mutant that does more or less whatever it wants: it is always active, favors the proliferation of cancerous cells, and can't be regulated.

And so every day I have to take GLIVEC, a tyrosine kinase inhibitor. It's like the **MUTANT GENE POLICE!**

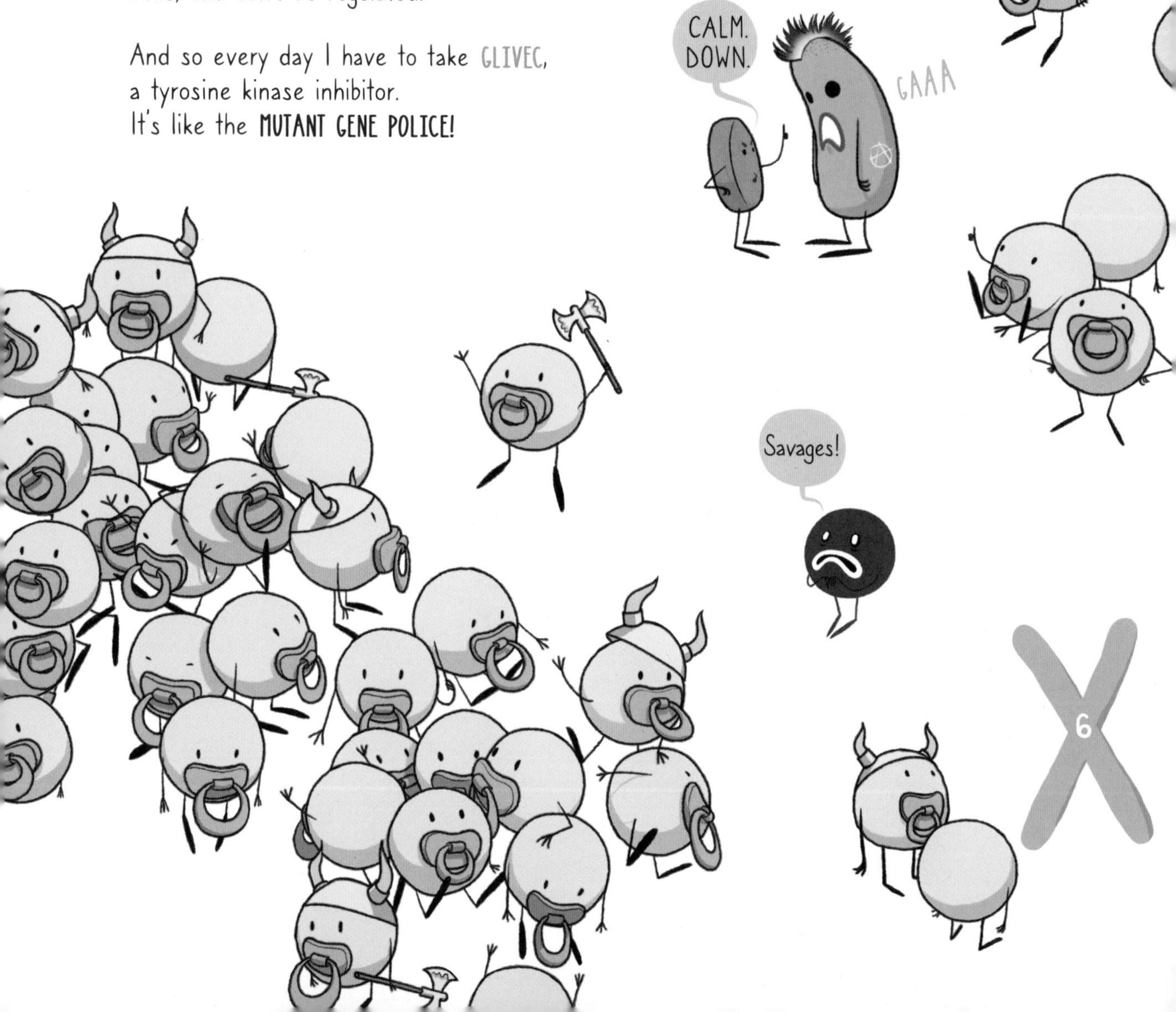
CALM. DOWN.
GAAA
Savages!
6

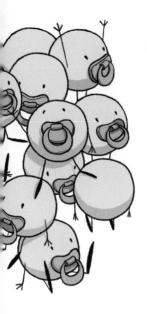

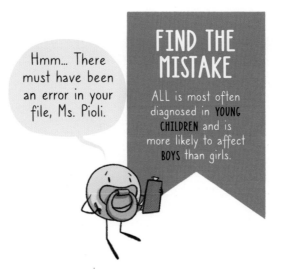

Hmm... There must have been an error in your file, Ms. Pioli.

FIND THE MISTAKE

ALL is most often diagnosed in **YOUNG CHILDREN** and is more likely to affect **BOYS** than girls.

THE GOOD NEWS is that it's not "genetic," in the sense that I won't transmit it to my children, and that my twin sister has no reason to have it, even though we have the same DNA.

8
9
I'm outta here!
Greetings from
NEW YORK
Greetings from
PHILADELPHIA
22
WELCOME TO Fabulous
LAS VEGAS
NEVADA

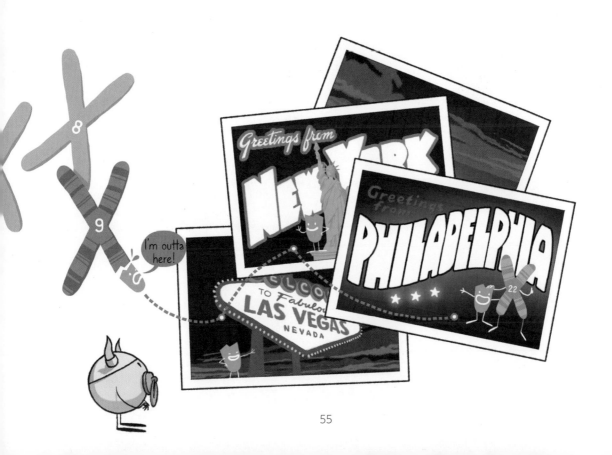

THE APLASIA FACTOR

Chemotherapy destroys my bone marrow cells, bringing their activity to a temporary halt.

- NO MORE RED BLOOD CELLS = anemia, fatigue.
- NO MORE PLATELETS = risk of hemorrhage.
- NO MORE WHITE BLOOD CELLS = risk of infection.

THIS IS WHAT'S CALLED APLASIA.

I have to wait until I'm out of this phase before I can leave the hospital. That's the reason my stay's been so long; the marrow can take several days/weeks to rebuild its stock of cells in sufficient quantity.

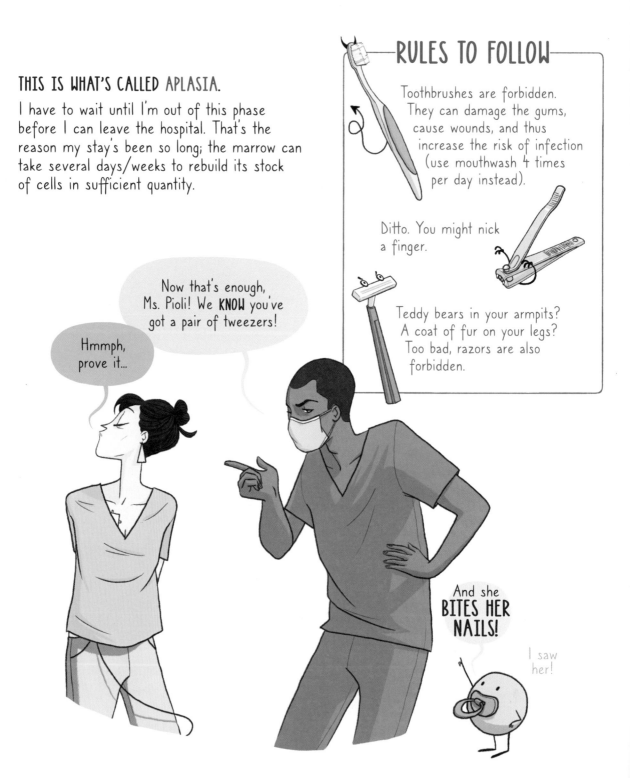

RULES TO FOLLOW

Toothbrushes are forbidden. They can damage the gums, cause wounds, and thus increase the risk of infection (use mouthwash 4 times per day instead).

Ditto. You might nick a finger.

Teddy bears in your armpits? A coat of fur on your legs? Too bad, razors are also forbidden.

Now that's enough, Ms. Pioli! We **KNOW** you've got a pair of tweezers!

Hmmph, prove it...

And she **BITES HER NAILS!**

I saw her!

My diet has been in **DEFENSE MODE** since the beginning, but now it's taken on a brand-new meaning: nothing raw (cooking kills bacteria), and the only fruits allowed are those with a peel (bananas and citrus, except for grapefruit, advised against when taking any kind of medication) in order to avoid any risk of infection.

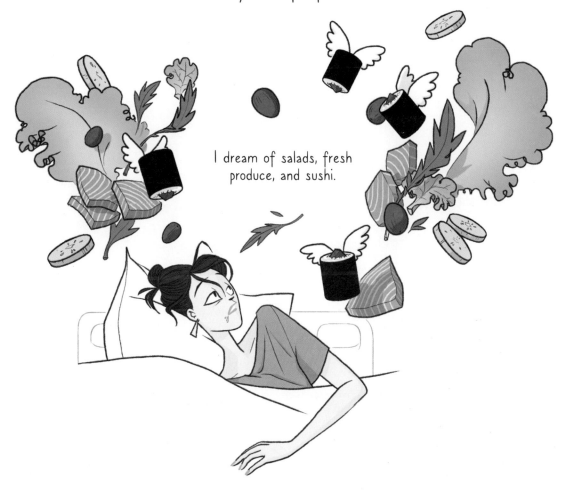

I dream of salads, fresh produce, and sushi.

BEFORE THE STORM

Shortly before going to the hospital, I had a conversation with my brother, Gabriel, which I remember very well.

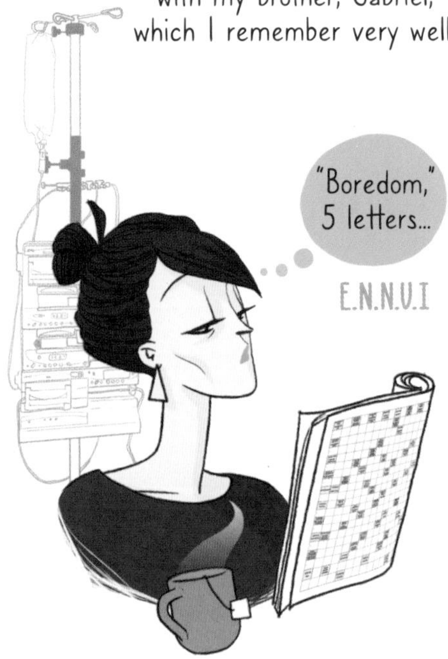
"Boredom," 5 letters...
E.N.N.U.I

While we were talking about my back problems, I explained to him that I was quite confident...

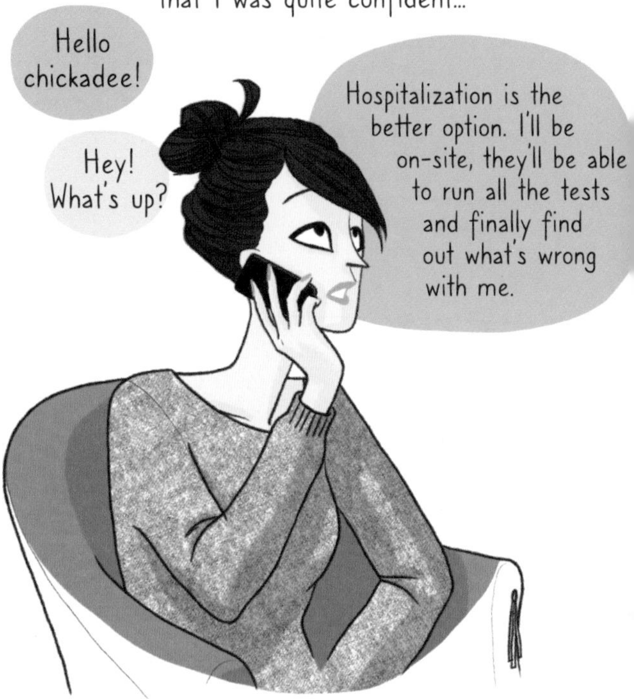
Hello chickadee!
Hey! What's up?
Hospitalization is the better option. I'll be on-site, they'll be able to run all the tests and finally find out what's wrong with me.

... but sometimes, I had "flashes of doubt," a growing anxiety that I did my best to ignore.

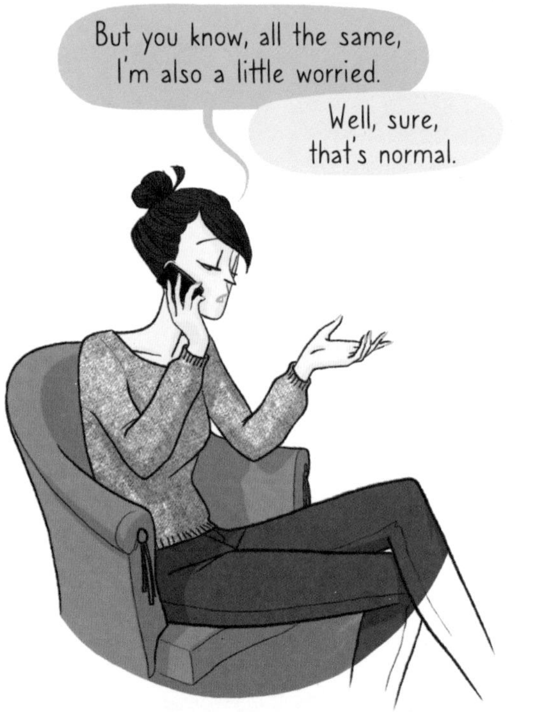
But you know, all the same, I'm also a little worried.
Well, sure, that's normal.

I was afraid that this "pre-hospital" period would be the last time I'd ever be happy again.

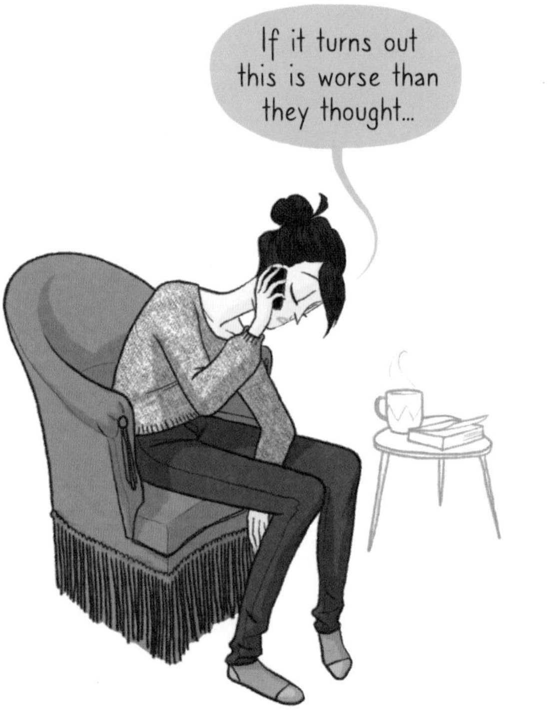
If it turns out this is worse than they thought...

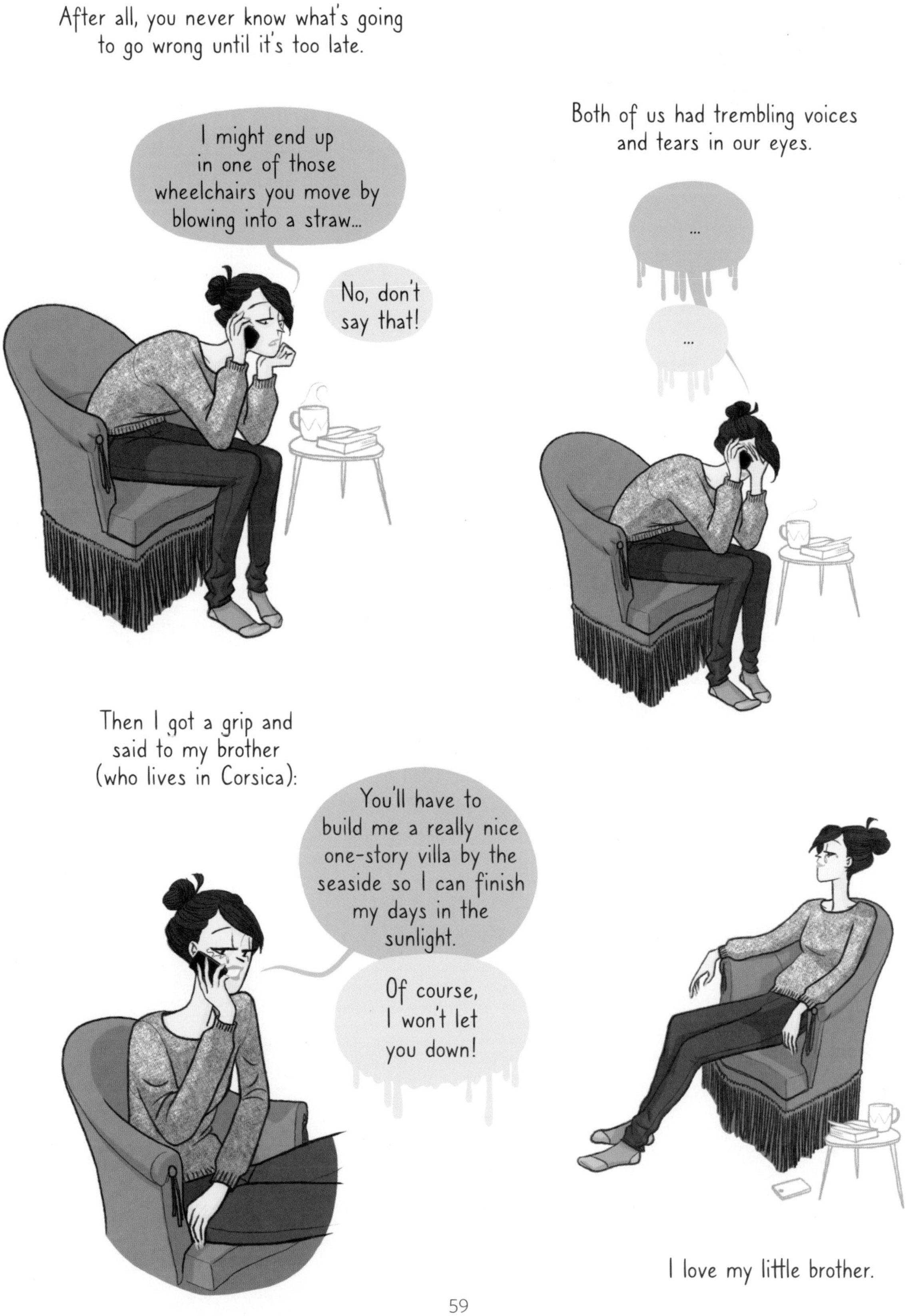
After all, you never know what's going to go wrong until it's too late.
I might end up in one of those wheelchairs you move by blowing into a straw...
No, don't say that!
Both of us had trembling voices and tears in our eyes.
...
...
Then I got a grip and said to my brother (who lives in Corsica):
You'll have to build me a really nice one-story villa by the seaside so I can finish my days in the sunlight.
Of course, I won't let you down!
I love my little brother.

A NEW WORLD

I used to feel like I was in control of my life, like I understood it.

JOURNEYS
LOVE

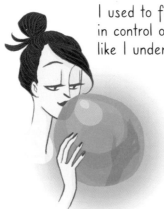

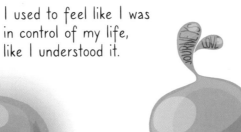

There were, of course, mishaps and surprises... But it always remained familiar, relatively certain.

WHATEVER THIS IS, IT'S SERIOUS

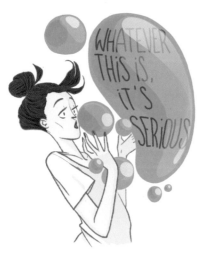

Now, I feel overwhelmed...

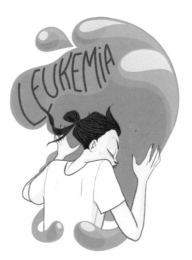

LEUKEMIA

...assaulted...

NOTHING IS CERTAIN ANYMORE

...submerged.

MARROW
BCR
BLASTS
PLATELETS
STEM
GROWTH FACTORS
CONDITIONING
MOLECULAR
CELLS
BLOOD COUNTS
BIOLOGY
CEREBROSPINAL LIQUID
NEUTROPENIA
VINCRISTINE
METHOTREXATE
ASPARAGINASE
MYELOPOIESIS
XANAX
THYMUS
TRANSPLANT
STEM CELLS
MYELOGRAM
CHEMO
CARDIAC

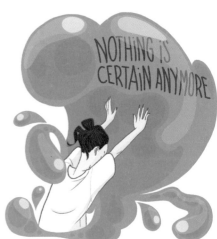

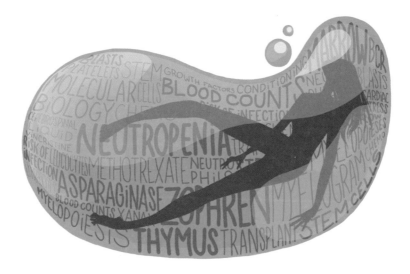

It's too much to absorb in too little time.

THE VIEW FROM OUTSIDE

"I came by the hospital. I saw you through the little window
in the door to your room. You were so skinny. I couldn't go in."
A friend told me that. It made me feel weird to realize that my sickness
was visible, that I looked sick and that it could push people away.

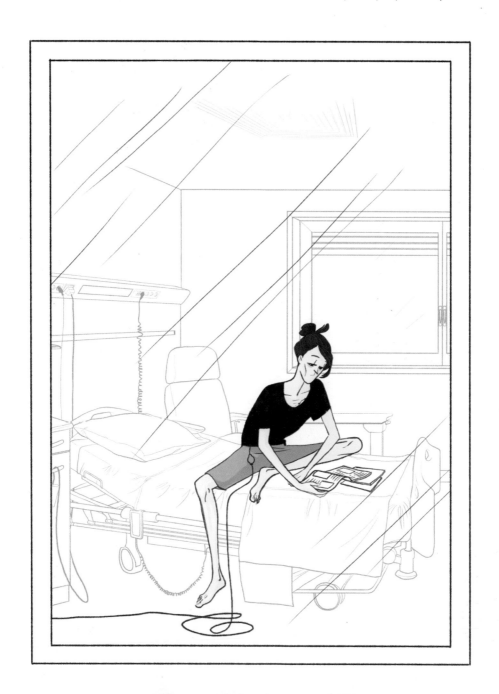

408

AND WHAT ABOUT MY BACK?

In addition to prescribing the chemo, they're trying to find the cause of my back pain, which is still there despite the corticosteroids. As for my sciatica, weirdly enough, I haven't had any pain even though things haven't let up for the past 6 months. Finally some good news!

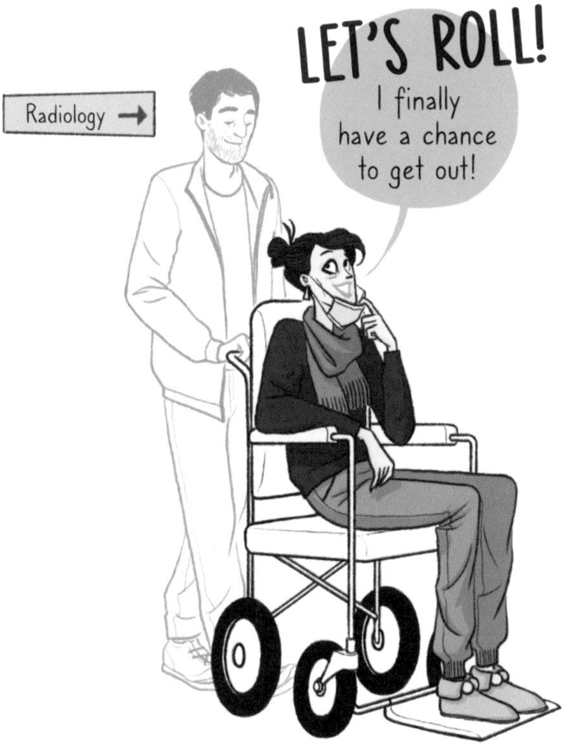
Radiology →
LET'S ROLL!
I finally have a chance to get out!

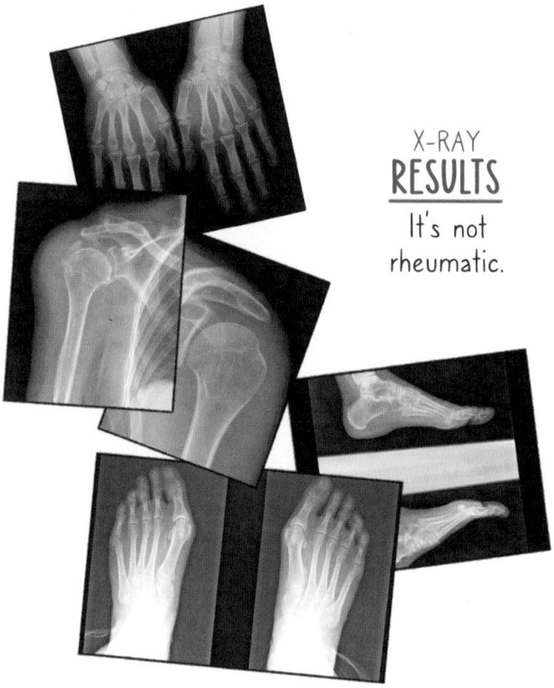

X-RAY

RESULTS

It's not rheumatic.

THE

SCINTIGRAPHY

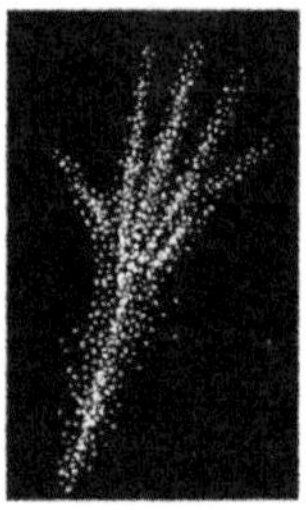

I'm injected with a radioactive substance that, after about fifteen minutes, attaches itself to my bones and reveals any potential lesions. On the monitor, during the exam, you can see your skeleton sparkle, made up of thousands of dots. It's rather pretty.

SCINTI

RESULTS

Inconclusive. A lot of the substance attached itself to my spinal cord, even though I don't have any lesions there, probably due to the chemotherapy.

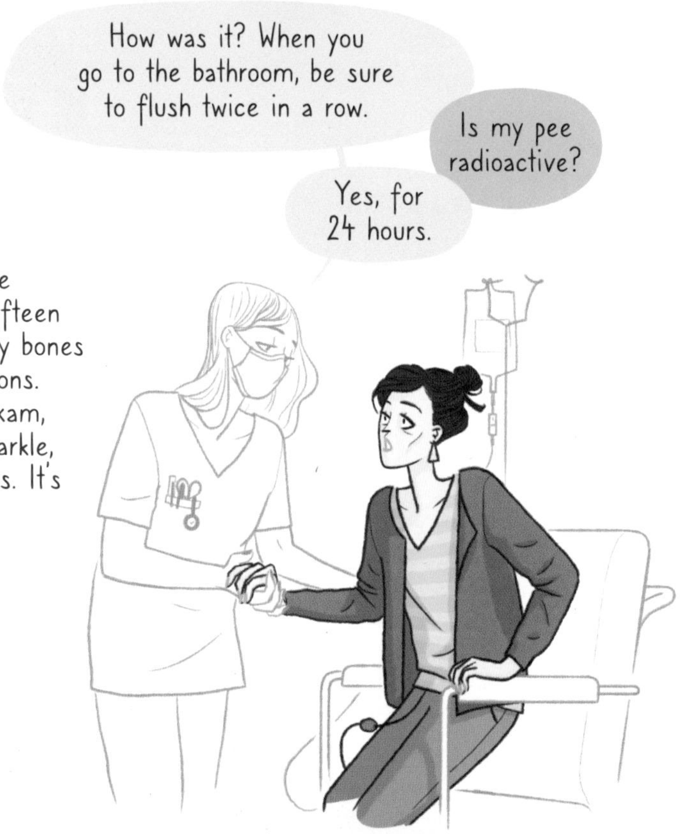
How was it? When you go to the bathroom, be sure to flush twice in a row.
Is my pee radioactive?
Yes, for 24 hours.

AND THE REST?

My stomach is rebelling by throwing up: it gets irritated and is taken by incredibly painful spasms. This lasts for some fifteen seconds, every 2 or 3 minutes.

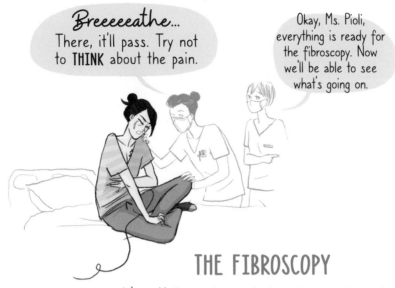

Breeeeeathe...
There, it'll pass. Try not to **THINK** about the pain.

Okay, Ms. Pioli, everything is ready for the fibroscopy. Now we'll be able to see what's going on.

THE FIBROSCOPY

<u>It's a Hollywood sound stage in my stomach...</u>

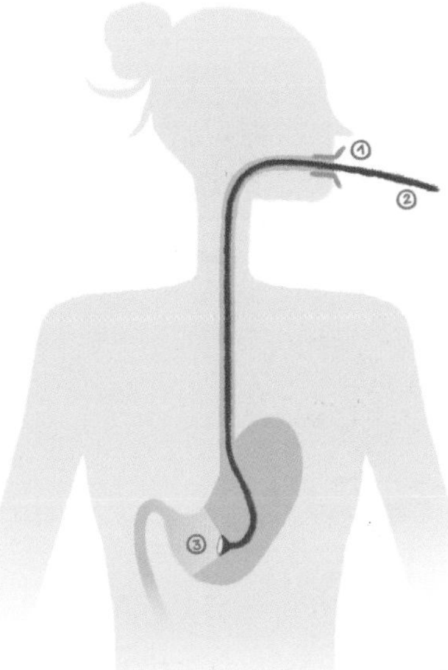

① Plastic thingy so I don't close my mouth.

② Pipe-camera that the gastroenterologist threads down my throat and into my stomach.
→ Retching

③ The camera shines a light. That makes sense, even though there's nothing to see. But it also blows out WIND! In order to inflate the stomach and smooth out folds to spot any potential lesions.

→ Where there's air in the stomach, there's also belching. For the 5 interminable minutes that the exam lasted, I burped/vomited air while drooling on myself, without being able to swallow, or throw up this fucking cable and make a break for it.

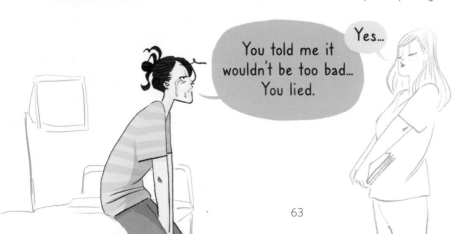

You told me it wouldn't be too bad... You lied.

Yes...

FIBRO
RESULTS

Stomach OK, the mystery remains, the pains stand alone.

FREE!

January 9—After being stuck in my room for almost a month and a half, I'm finally over my aplasia and out of the hospital! The dietitian stops by to "brief" me before I leave...

BACTERIA

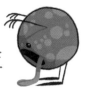

RULES TO FOLLOW AT HOME

to keep out of the hospital,
for now.

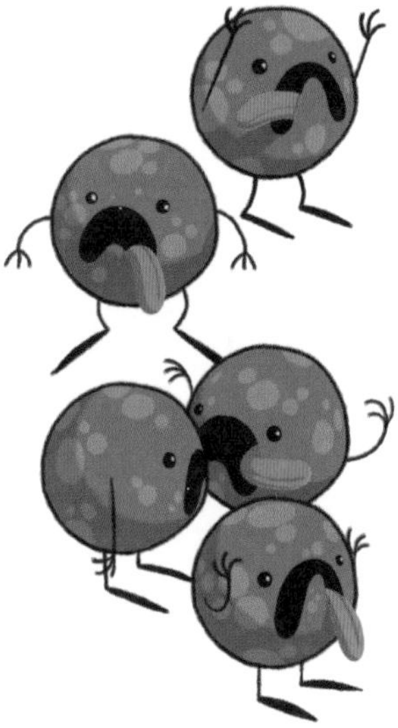

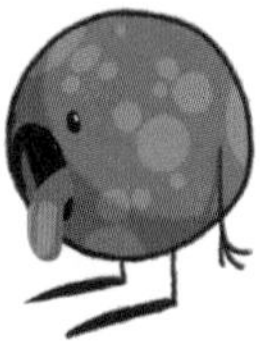

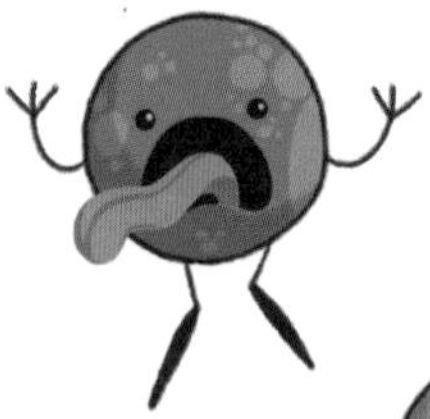

Disinfect kitchenware and food containers.

—

No subways, pools, or movie theaters
(places where people congregate).

—

No raw meat (so long, tartare!)
or fish (so long, sushi!!!).
Only cooked foods.

—

Wash vegetables in vinegared water
if you want to eat them raw.

—

"Once it's opened, you have to eat it!"
Applies to cakes, chips, candy, etc.

—

Disinfect the fridge every 15 days.

—

No leftovers.

—

No food from deli counters,
only pre-packaged.

—

No charcuterie or cheeses made
from unpasteurized milk.

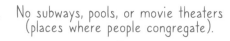

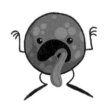

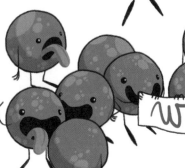

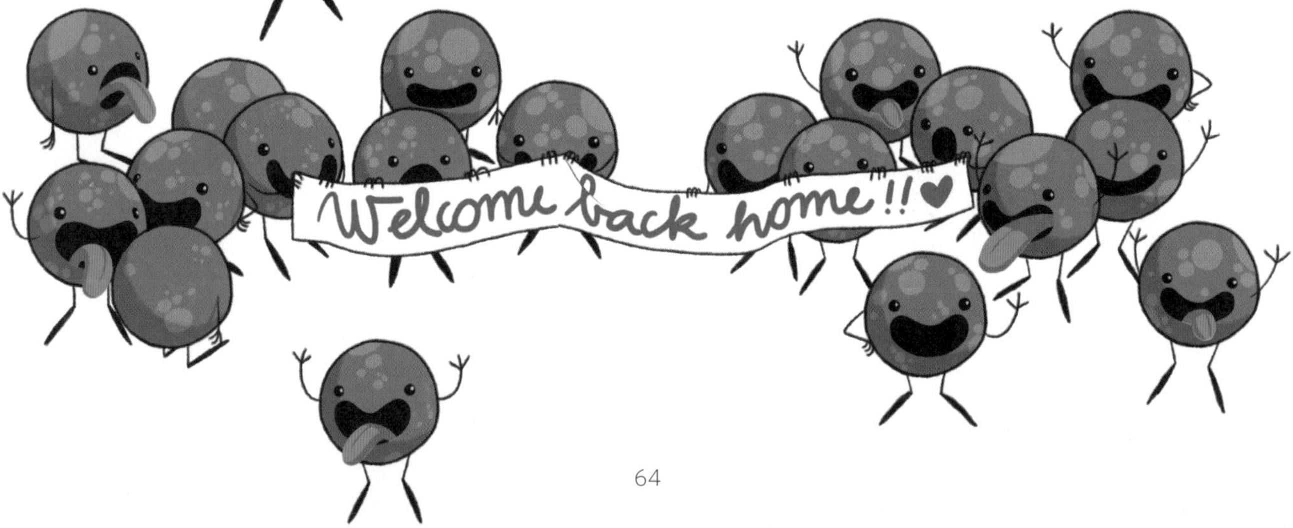

Welcome back home !!♥

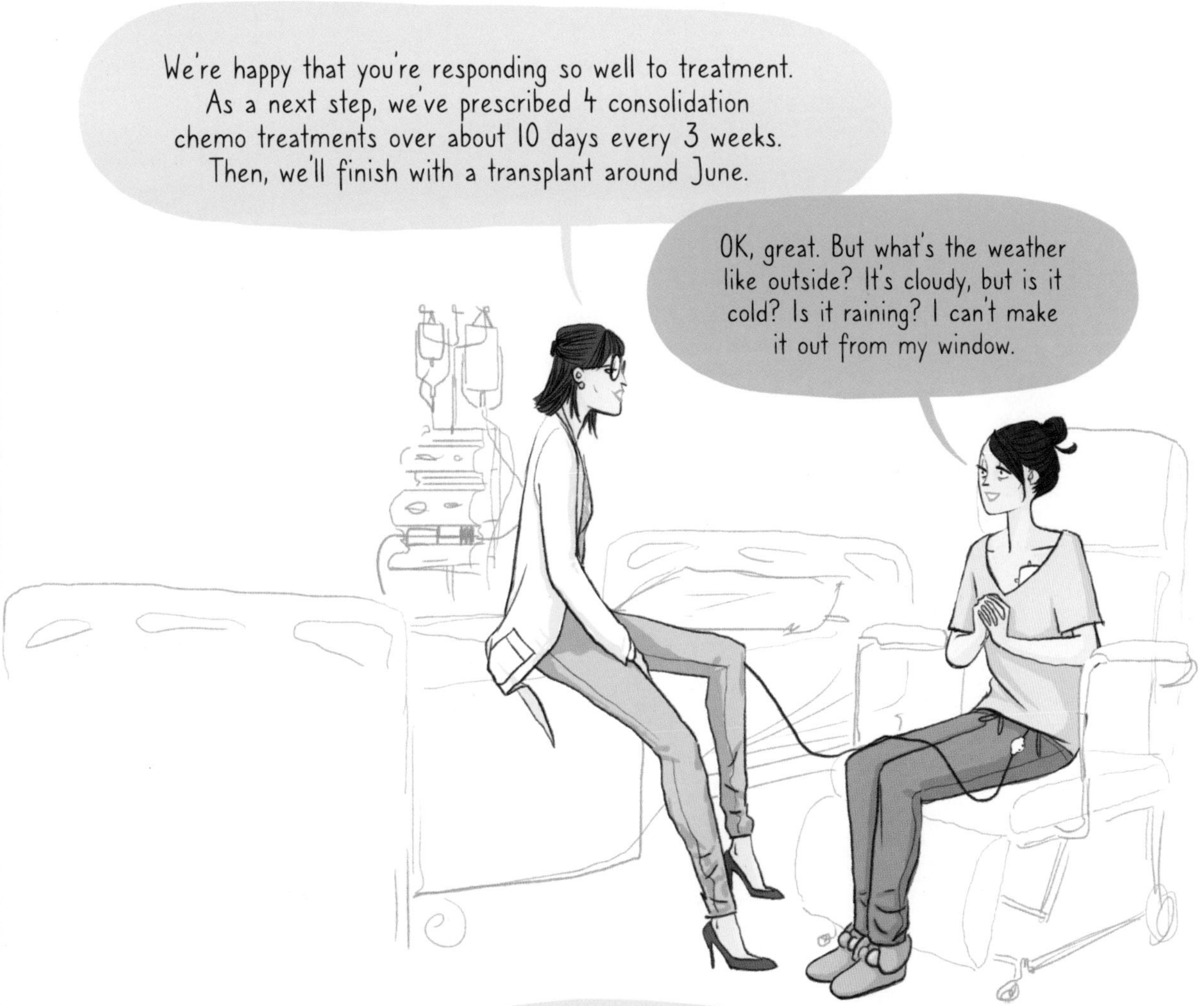
We're happy that you're responding so well to treatment. As a next step, we've prescribed 4 consolidation chemo treatments over about 10 days every 3 weeks. Then, we'll finish with a transplant around June.
OK, great. But what's the weather like outside? It's cloudy, but is it cold? Is it raining? I can't make it out from my window.

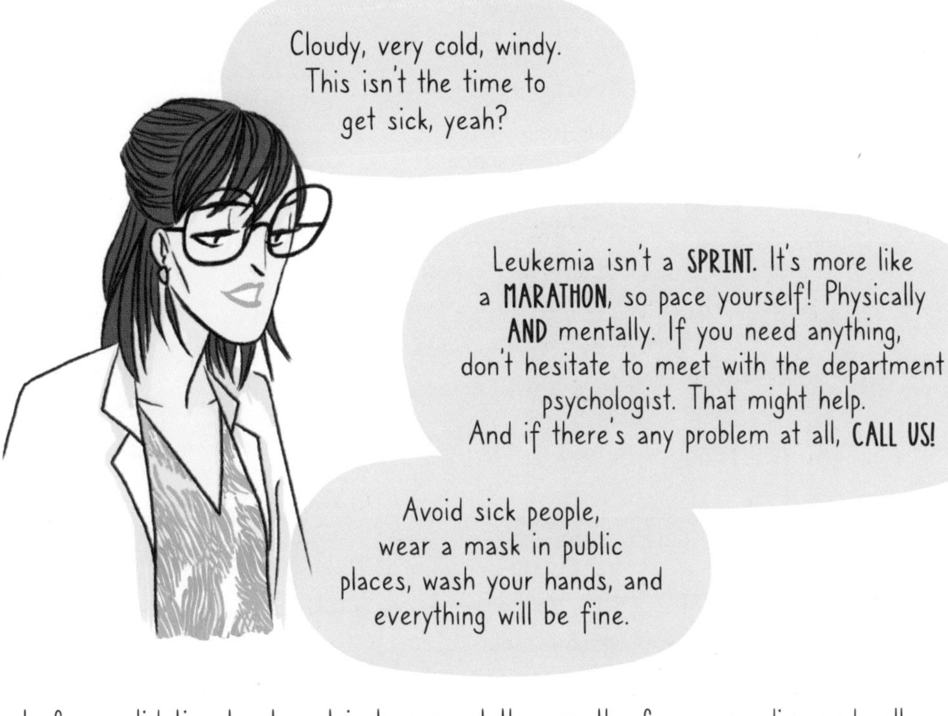
Cloudy, very cold, windy. This isn't the time to get sick, yeah?
Leukemia isn't a SPRINT. It's more like a MARATHON, so pace yourself! Physically AND mentally. If you need anything, don't hesitate to meet with the department psychologist. That might help. And if there's any problem at all, CALL US!
Avoid sick people, wear a mask in public places, wash your hands, and everything will be fine.

*The goal of consolidation treatment is to prevent the growth of any new diseased cells.

A PROBLEM...

My weight loss hasn't stopped, and now I weigh 88 pounds. I had avoided nasogastric feeding since I was still above the malnutrition threshold. But I've lost 40 pounds total! And I didn't realize what this meant, besides the "lost volume," until it was time to leave.

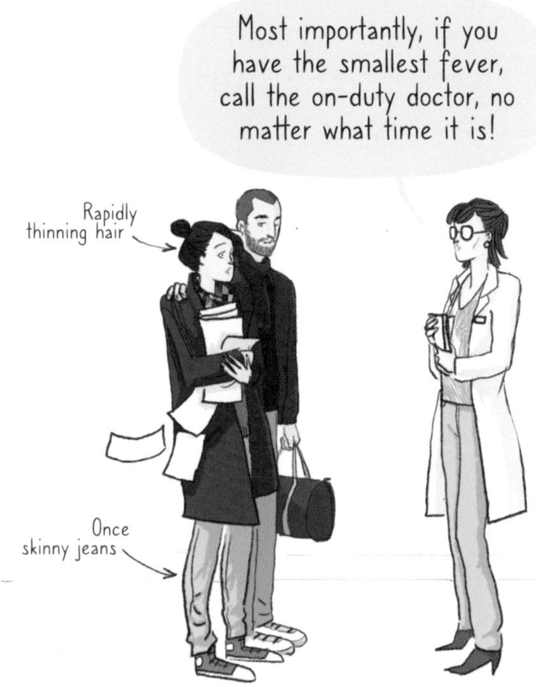
Most importantly, if you have the smallest fever, call the on-duty doctor, no matter what time it is!
Rapidly thinning hair
Once skinny jeans

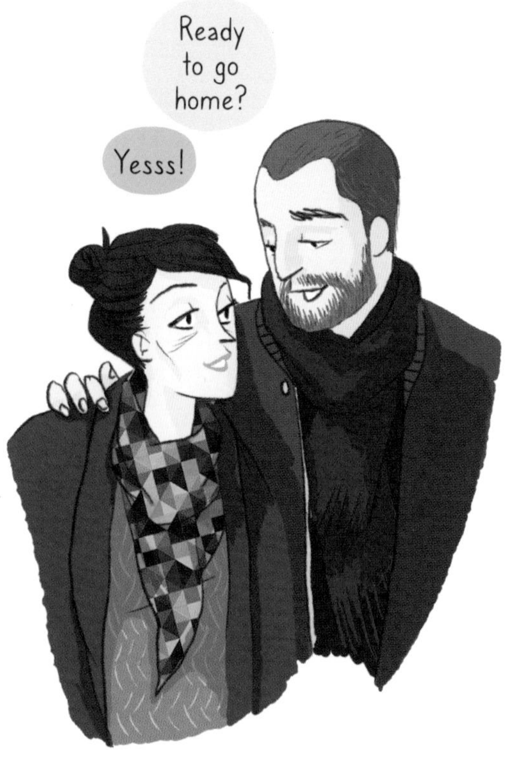
Ready to go home?
Yesss!

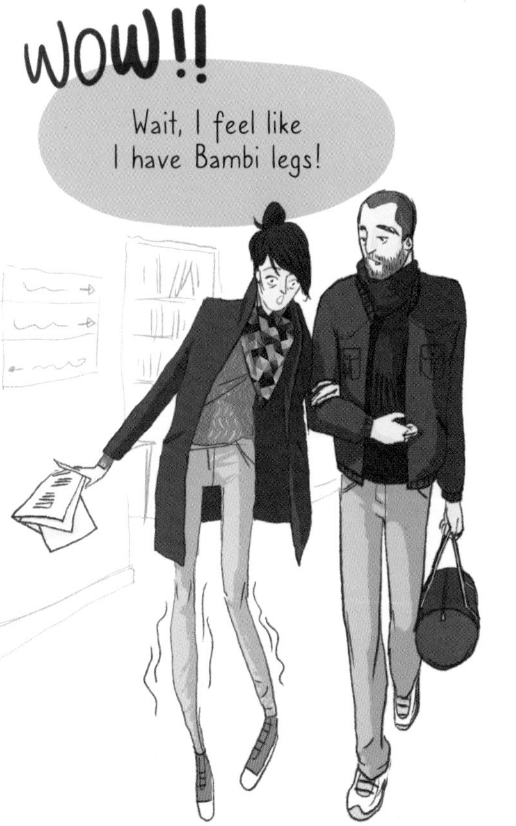
WOW!!
Wait, I feel like I have Bambi legs!

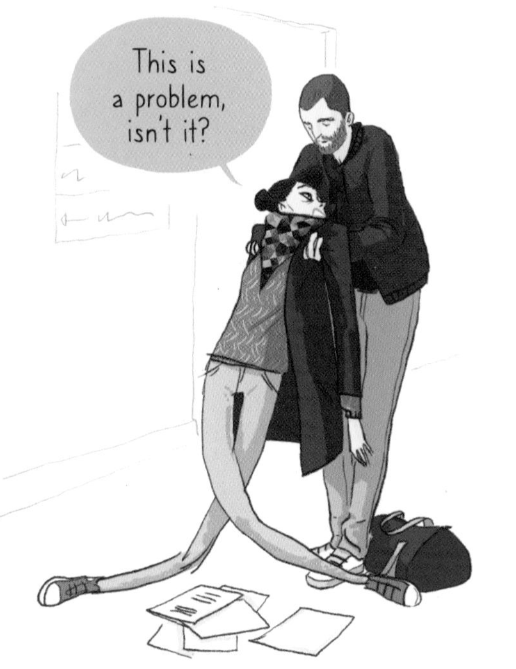
This is a problem, isn't it?

Well, I'm exaggerating. But only a little!

This, unfortunately, wasn't the only problem. It was also the day they took hostages at the kosher supermarket at the Porte de Vincennes. I had been following the *Charlie Hebdo* murders that'd happened 2 days before my hospital bubble, but now it was becoming all too real, since I was leaving my protective bubble and setting foot back into "real" life in a rather brutal manner.

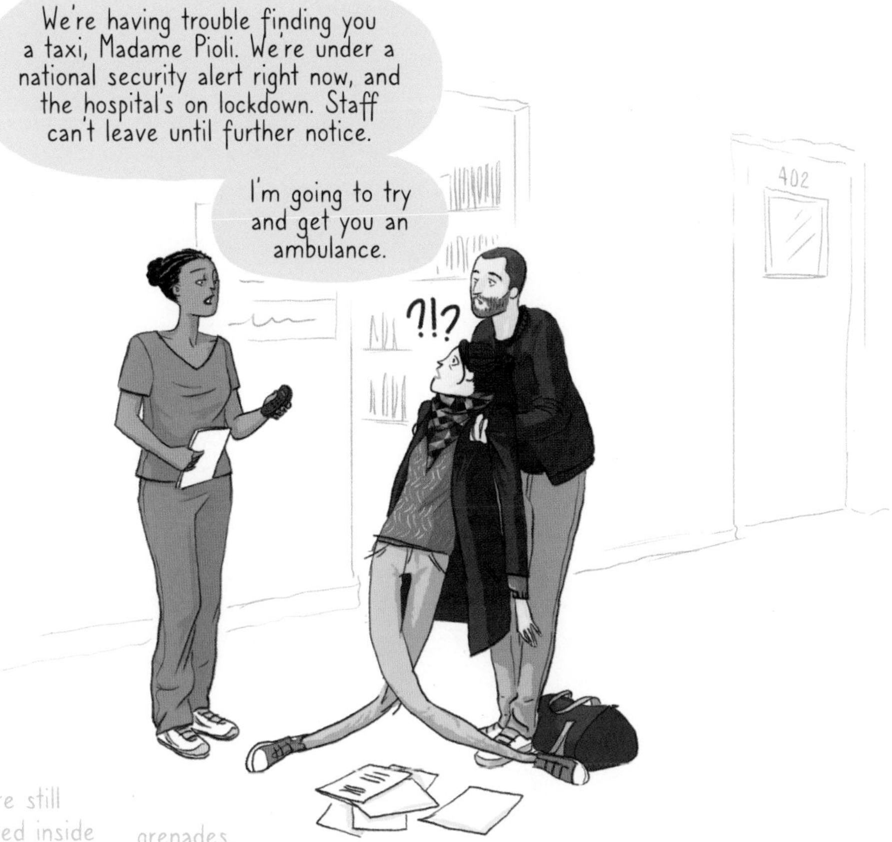

We're having trouble finding you a taxi, Madame Pioli. We're under a national security alert right now, and the hospital's on lockdown. Staff can't leave until further notice.
I'm going to try and get you an ambulance.
?!?
402

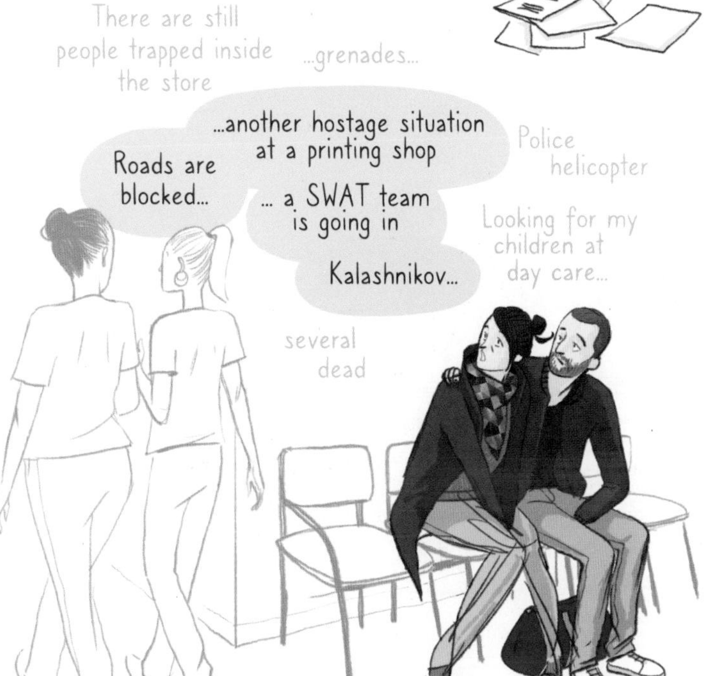

There are still people trapped inside the store
...grenades...
...another hostage situation at a printing shop
Roads are blocked...
... a SWAT team is going in
Police helicopter
Looking for my children at day care...
Kalashnikov...
several dead

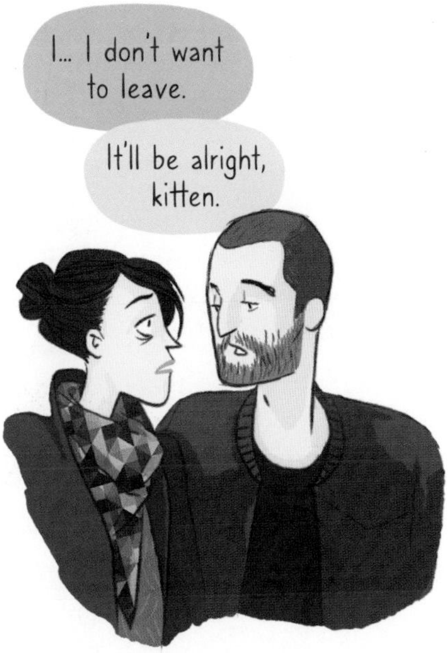

I... I don't want to leave.
It'll be alright, kitten.

After waiting for several hours, someone finds an ambulance to take me home. Being at last outside feels strange. The air is cold, and I can feel the wind on my face. It's raining and the sky is gray. And this strangeness is reinforced by the police surrounding the hospital, the tense atmosphere, the seemingly deserted streets, and my fearful anxiety. It's happening, I'm outside, and there's nothing to protect me. From illness, bacteria, or terrorists. Everything is jumbled together. I feel abandoned and on my own.

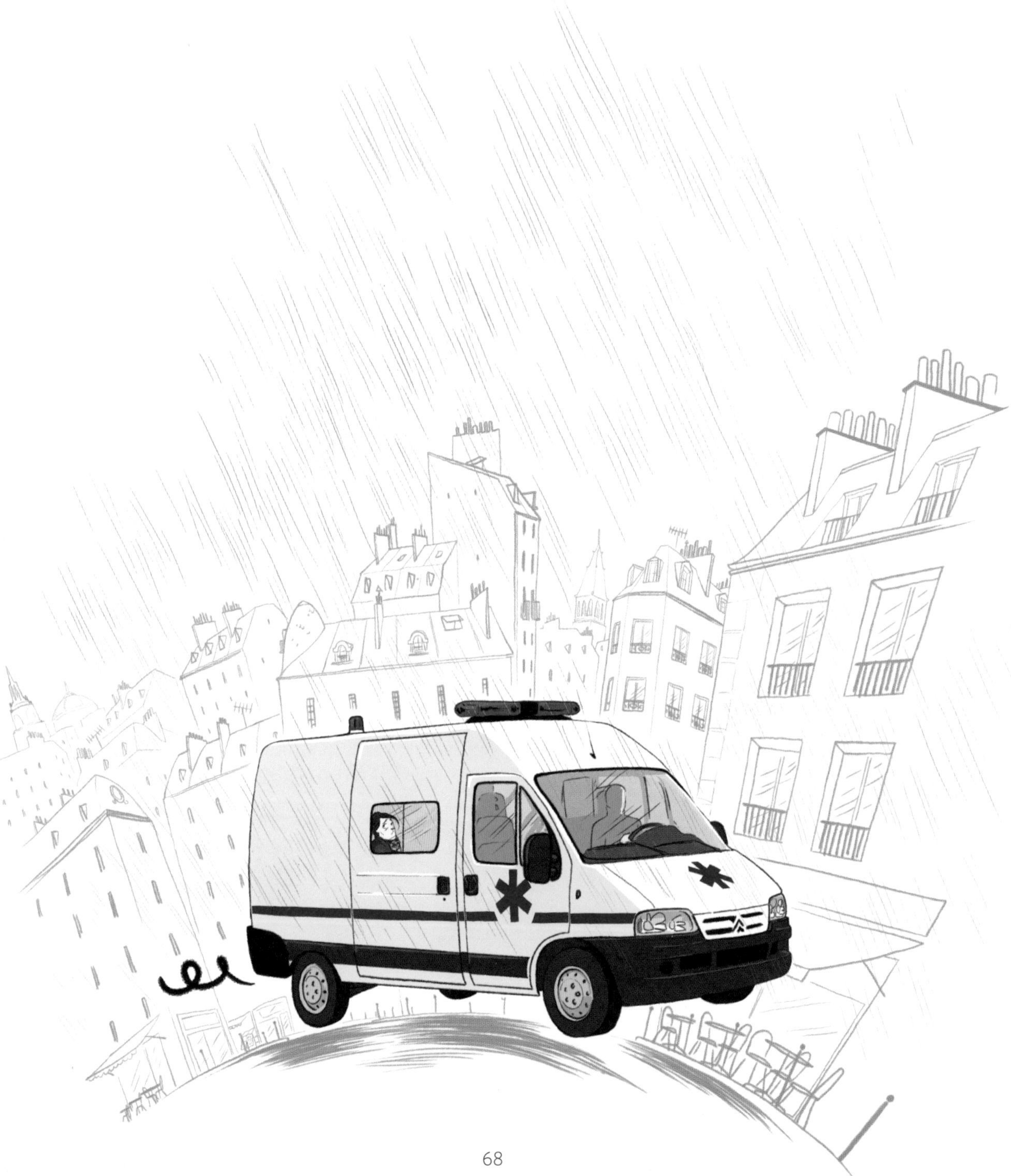

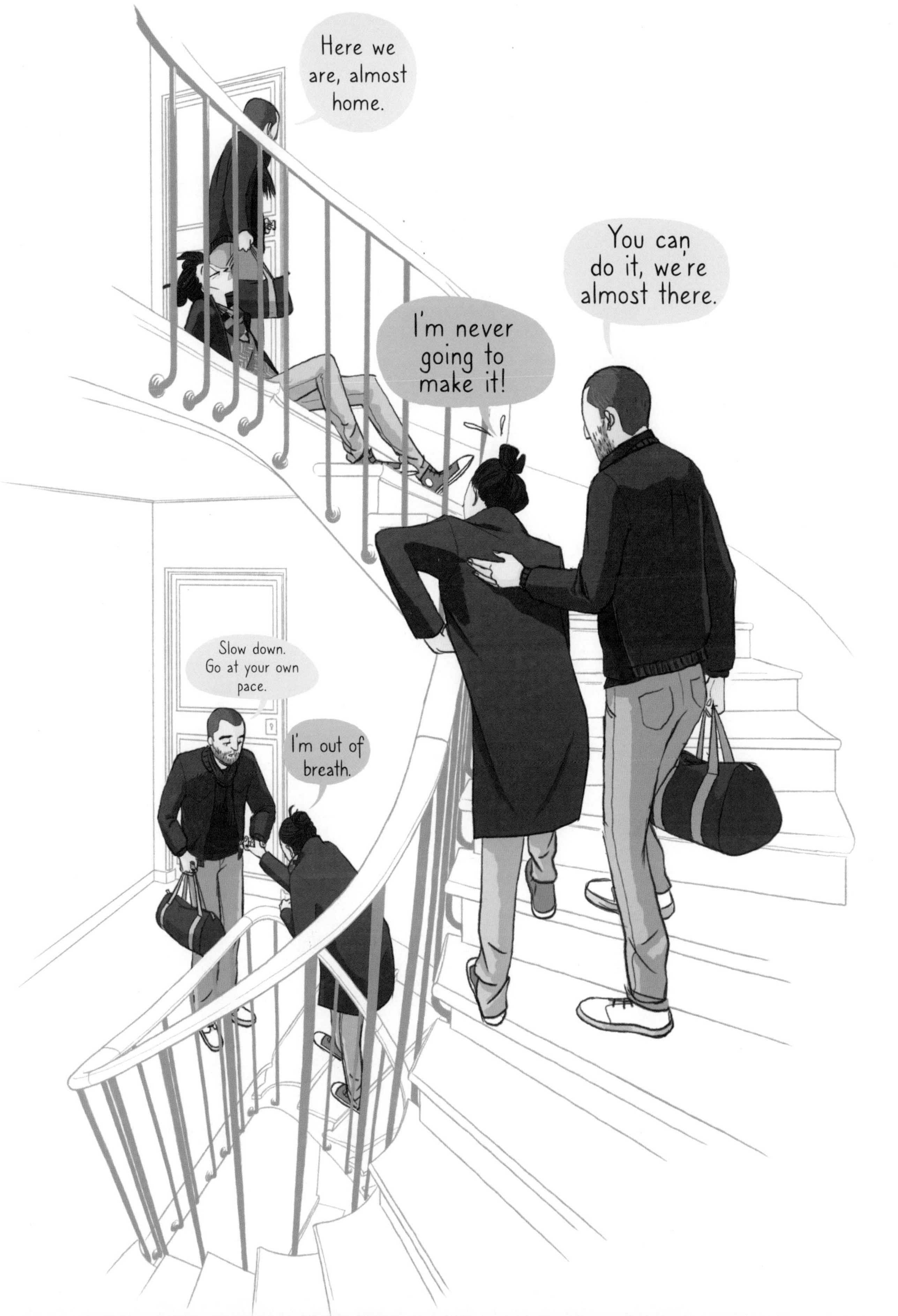
Here we are, almost home.
You can do it, we're almost there.
I'm never going to make it!
Slow down. Go at your own pace.
I'm out of breath.

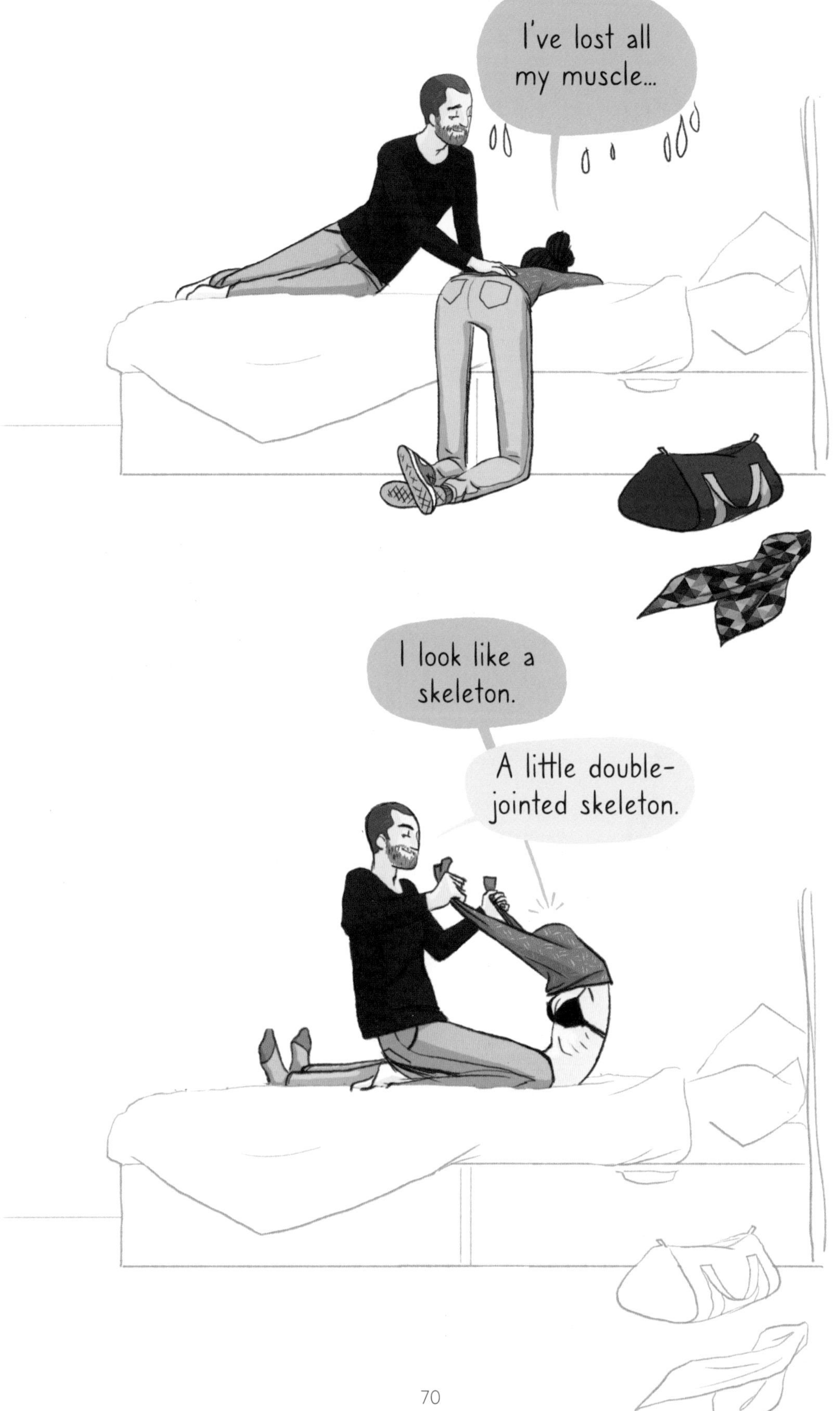
I've lost all my muscle...
I look like a skeleton.
A little double-jointed skeleton.

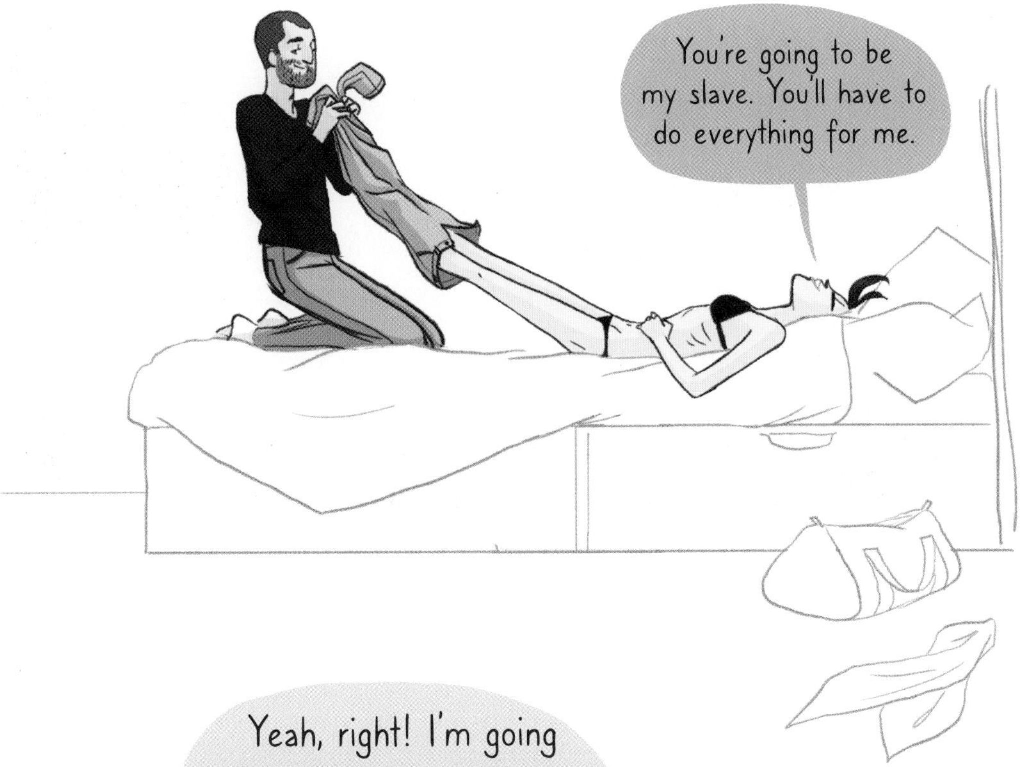
You're going to be my slave. You'll have to do everything for me.

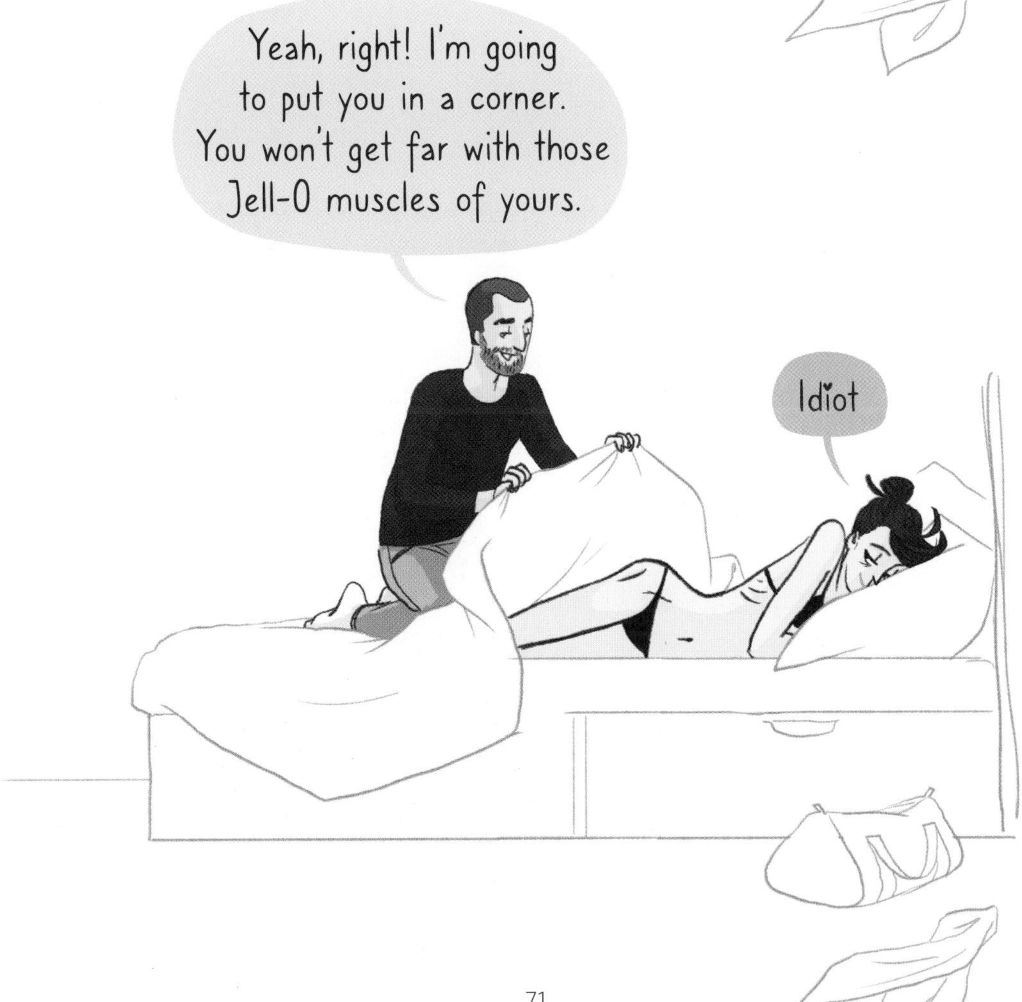
Yeah, right! I'm going to put you in a corner. You won't get far with those Jell-O muscles of yours.
Idiot

The first few days are hard. I'm still nauseated by the thought of eating. I guess my stomach must have shrunk. But I start to get cravings, sort of like a pregnant woman.

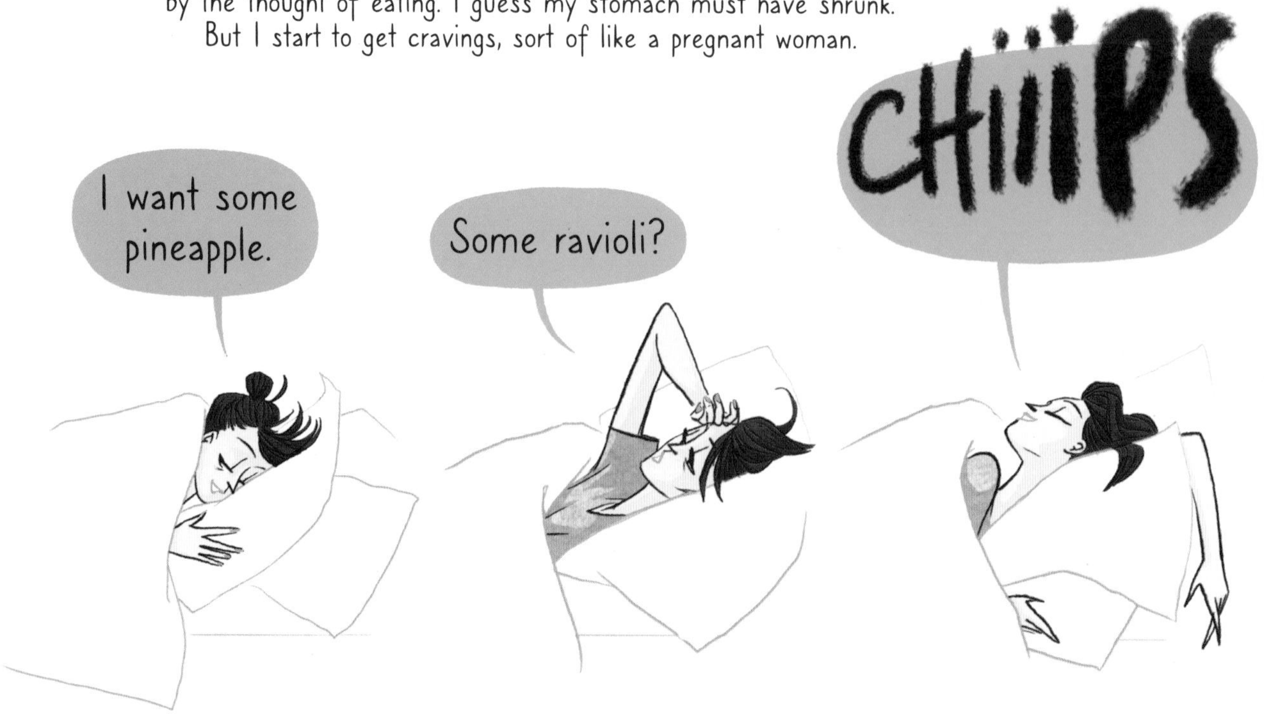
I want some pineapple.
Some ravioli?
CHIIIPS

And then I realize that I've been "conditioned." From now on, hospital = vomit.

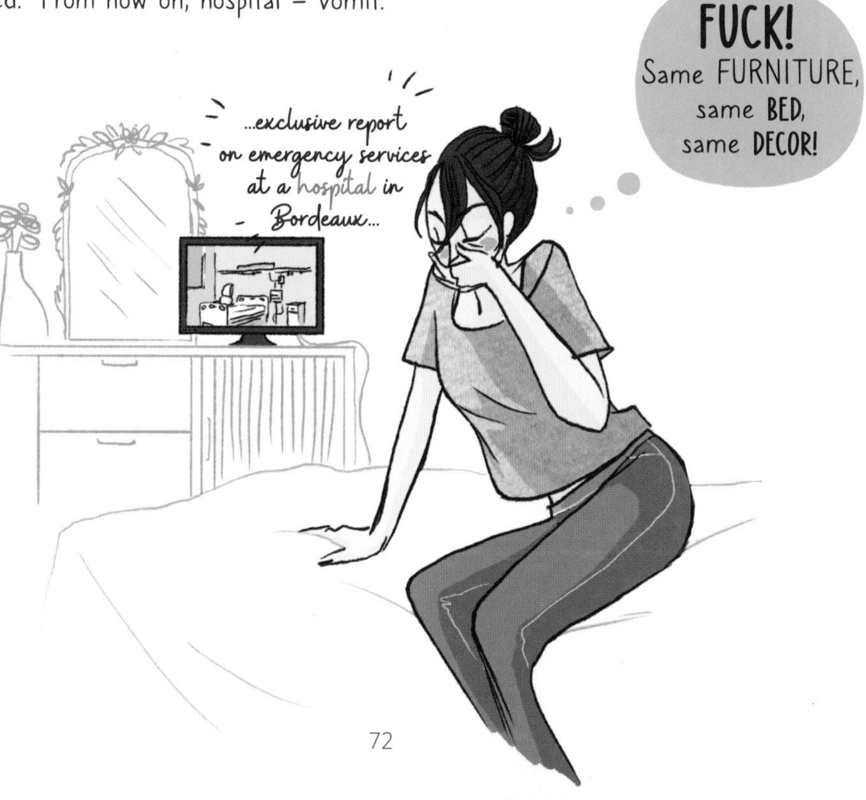
...exclusive report on emergency services at a hospital in Bordeaux...
FUCK! Same FURNITURE, same BED, same DECOR!

I've also become more sensitive to certain things.

The smell of casseroles...

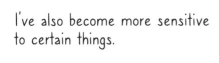

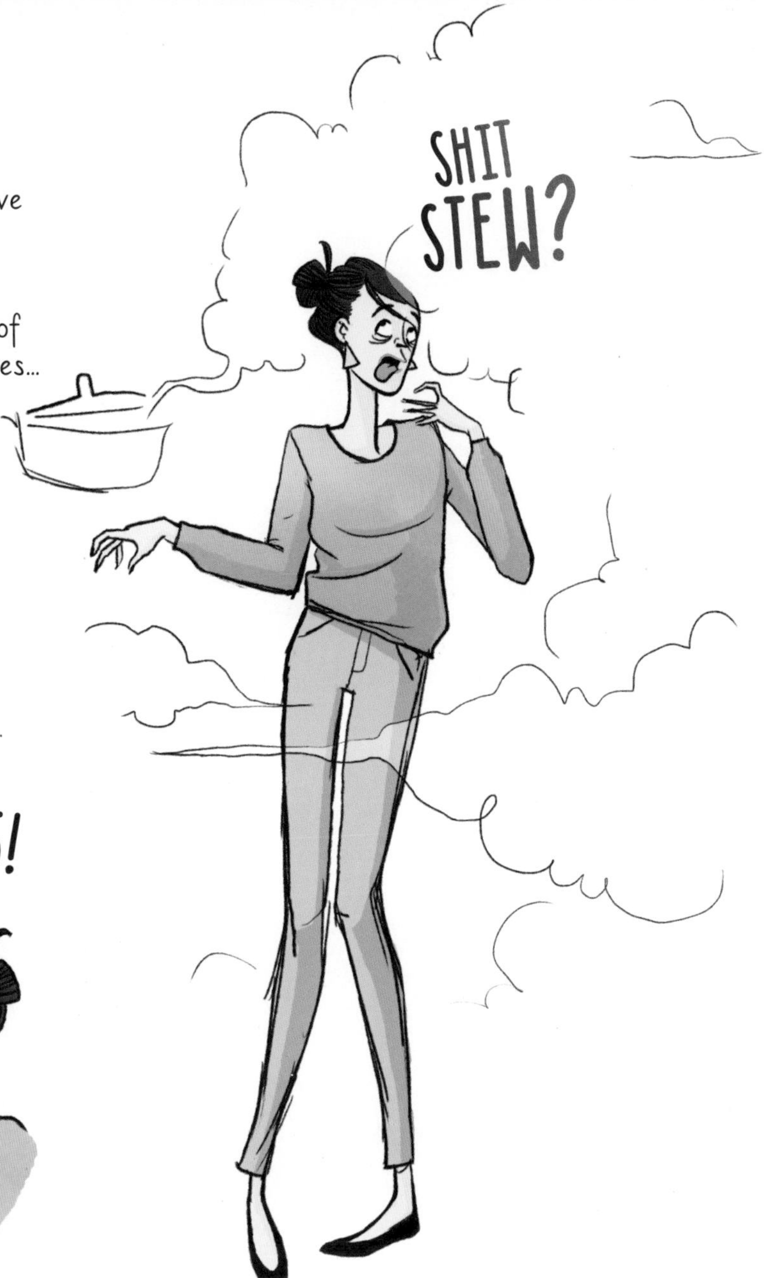
SHIT STEW?

...people's perfumes...

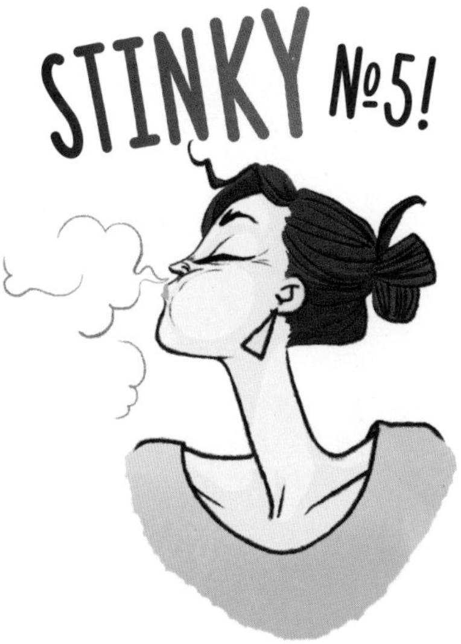
STINKY №5!

Even **WATER** makes me want to throw up, since I now associate it with taking medications.

I trick myself with Coke and flavored or sparkling waters, but they're still hard to drink.

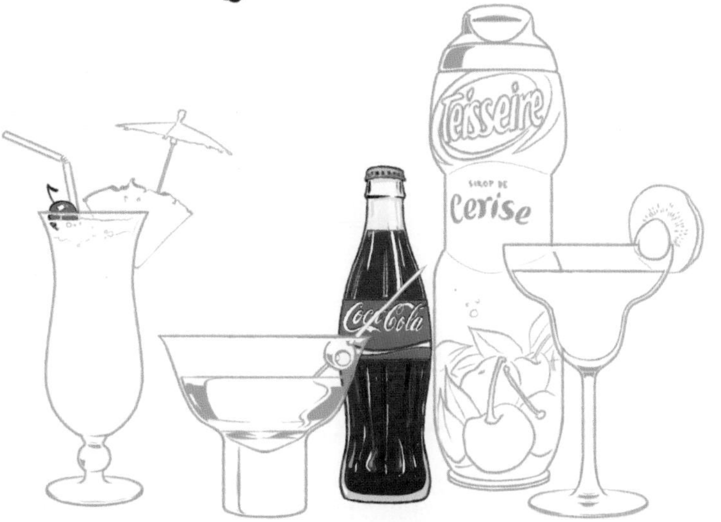
Teisseire
SIROP DE
Cerise
Coca-Cola

THIS NUMBER IS NO LONGER IN SERVICE

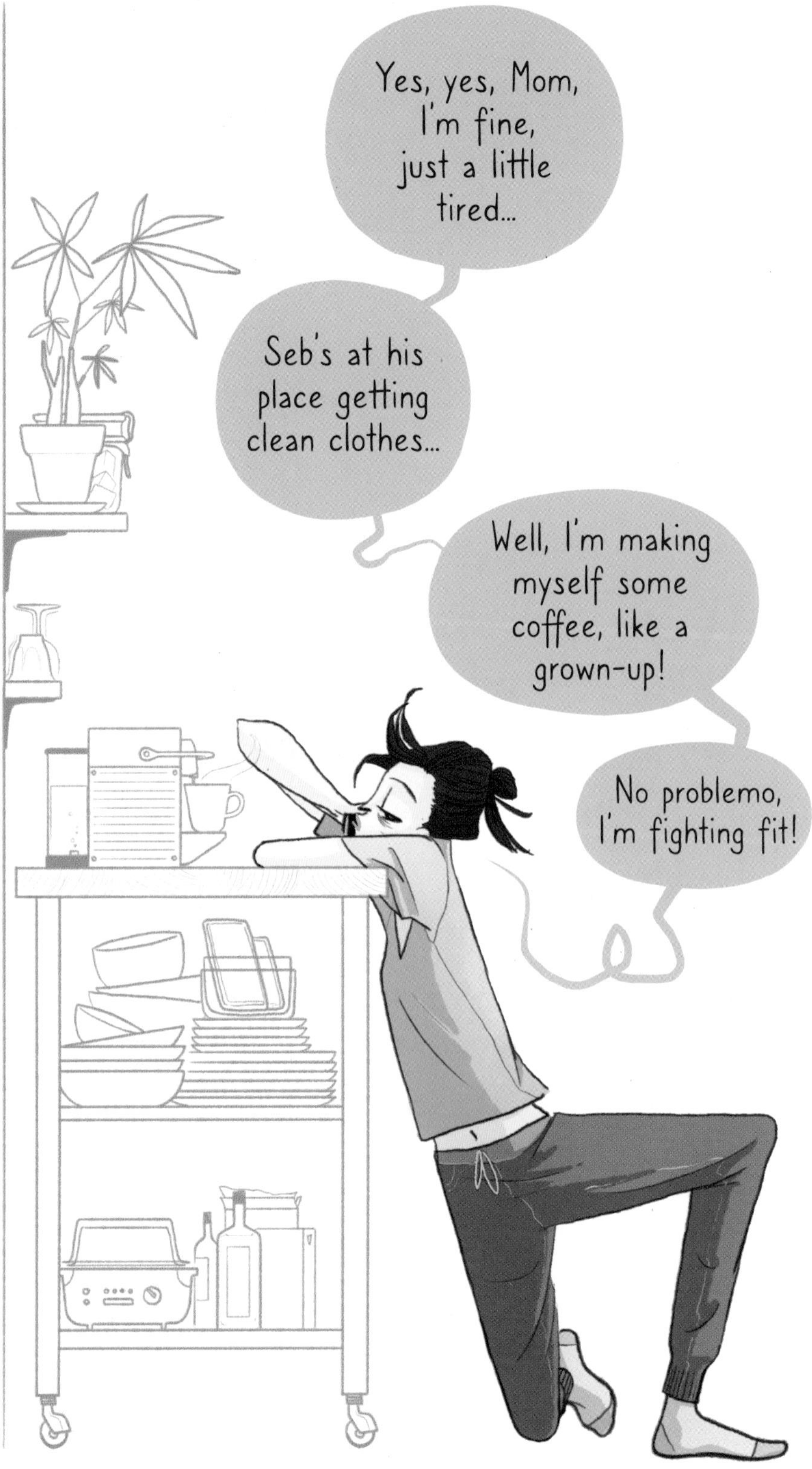
Yes, yes, Mom, I'm fine, just a little tired...
Seb's at his place getting clean clothes...
Well, I'm making myself some coffee, like a grown-up!
No problemo, I'm fighting fit!

I haven't been feeling all that great lately. I don't think I've ever been so tired in all my life. My relief at finally being back home has transformed into the need to hibernate.

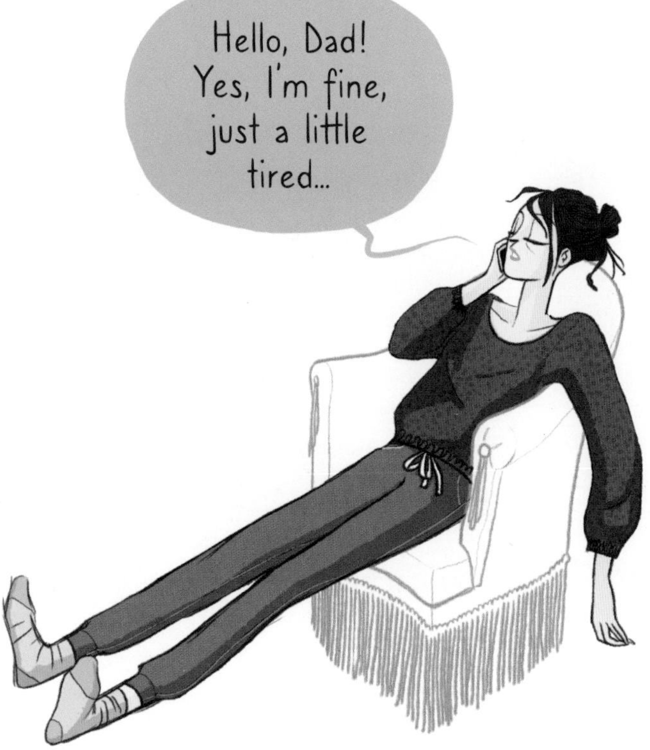
Hello, Dad! Yes, I'm fine, just a little tired...

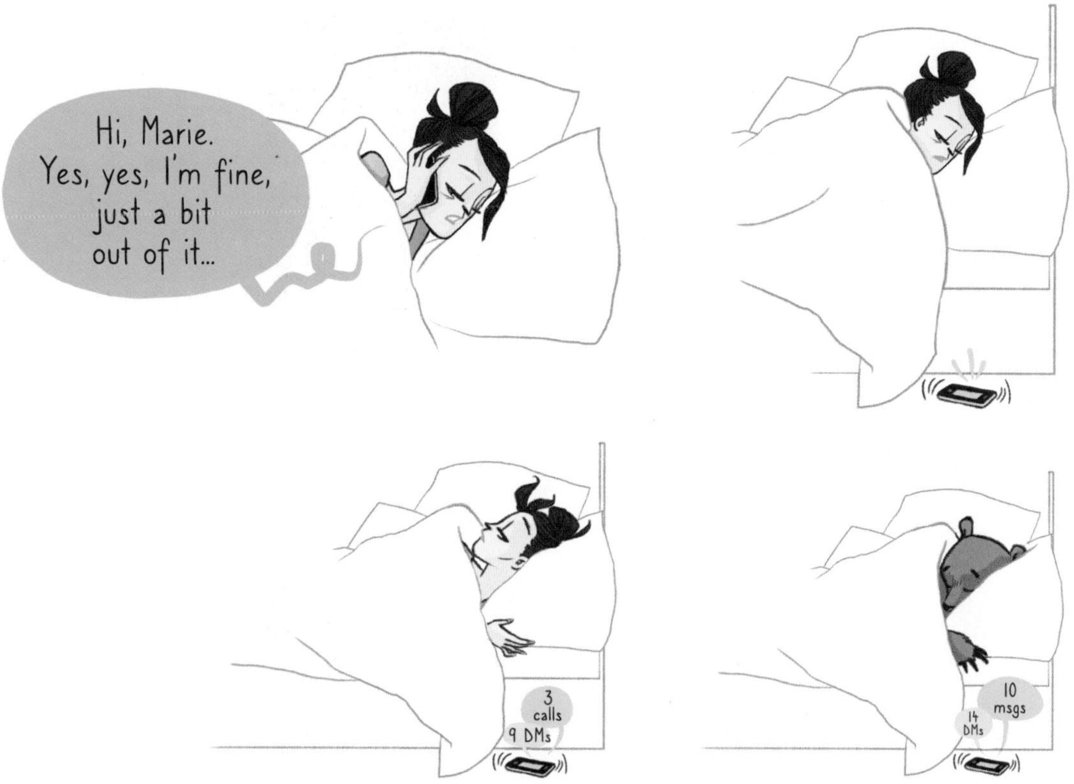
Hi, Marie. Yes, yes, I'm fine, just a bit out of it...
3 calls
9 DMs
10 msgs
14 DMs

I'm also having trouble concentrating (what day is it?) or staying upright (I sit in the shower to wash myself so I don't pass out).

MICROBES

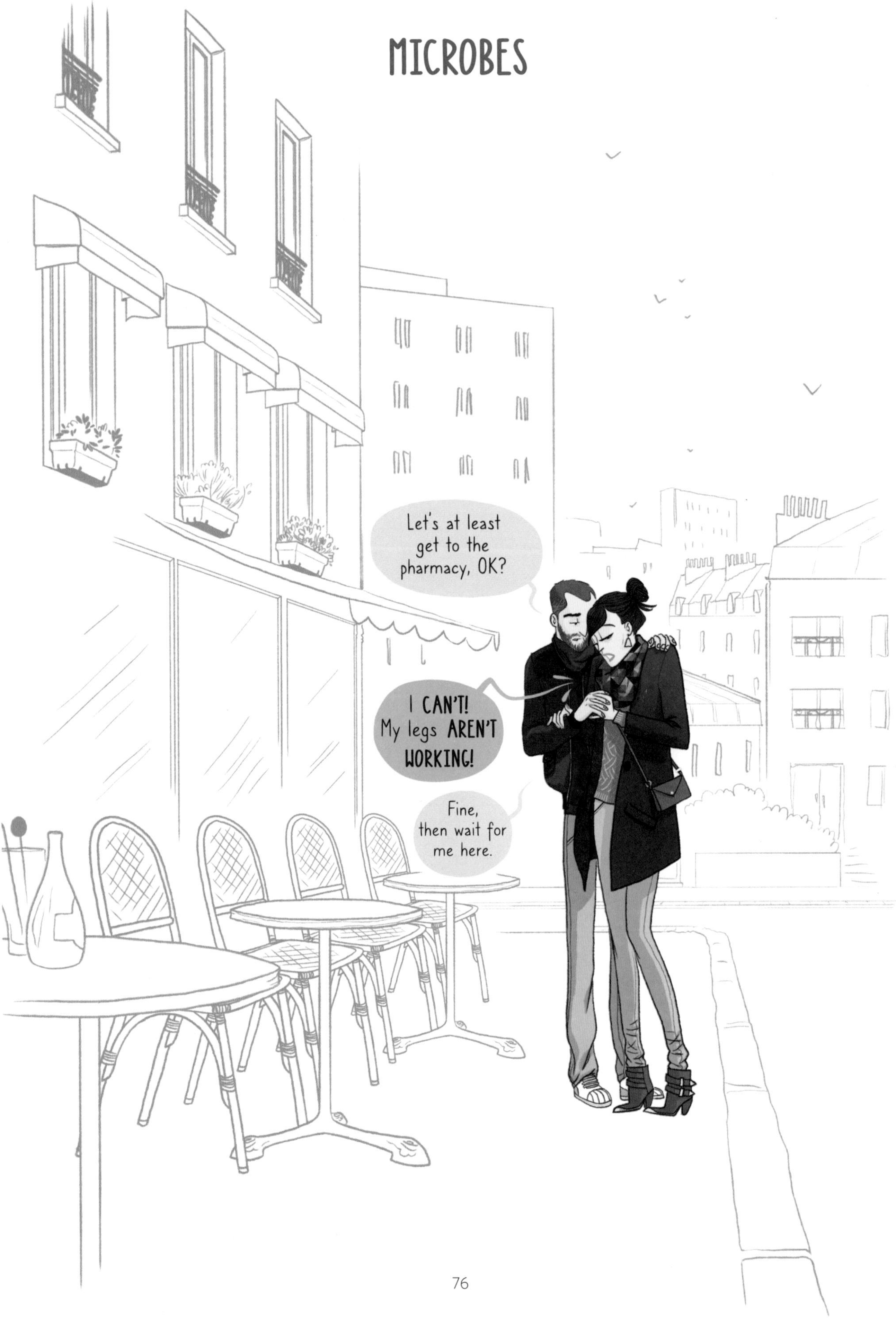

Let's at least get to the pharmacy, OK?
I CAN'T! My legs AREN'T WORKING!
Fine, then wait for me here.

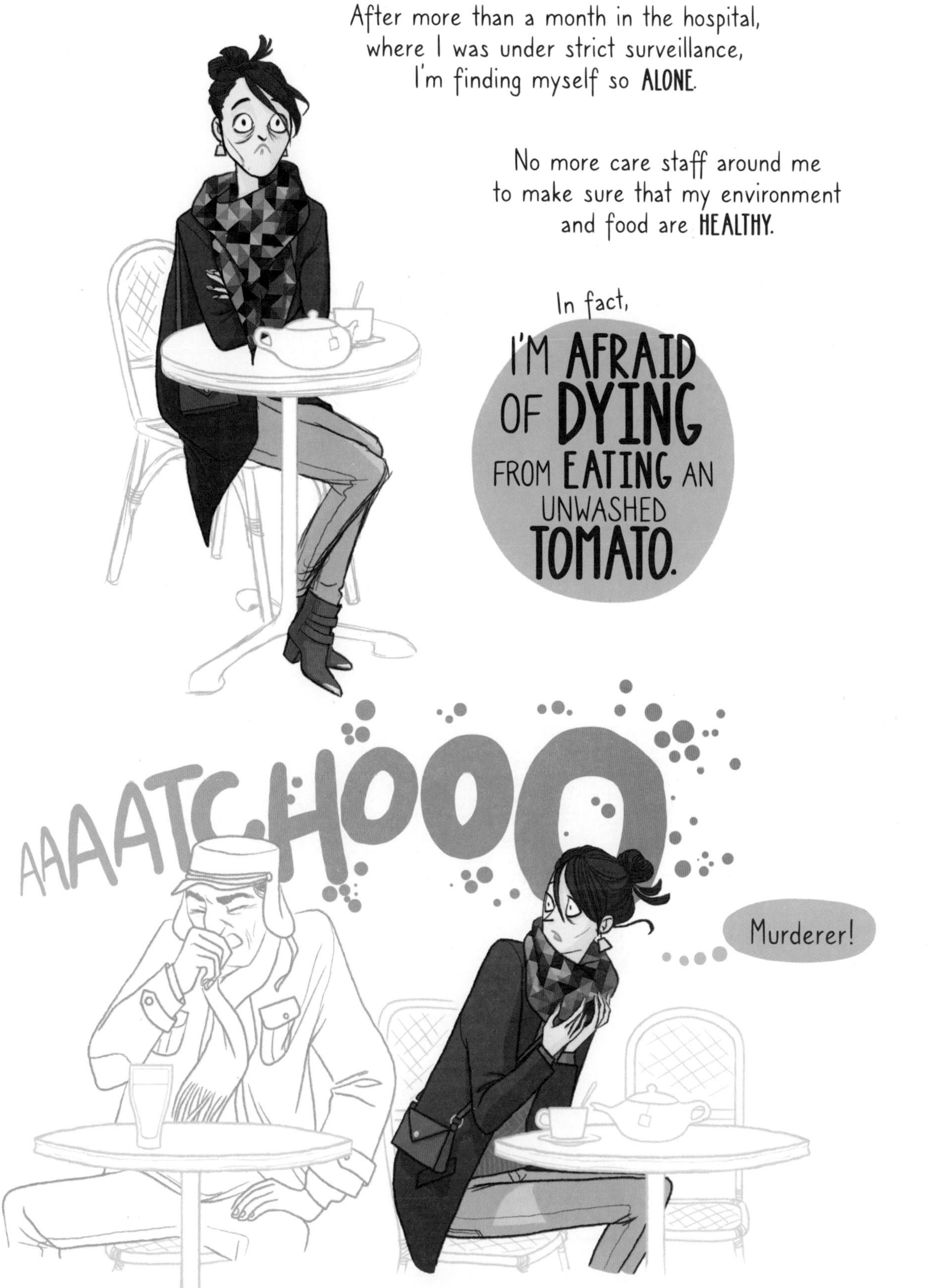
After more than a month in the hospital, where I was under strict surveillance, I'm finding myself so ALONE.
No more care staff around me to make sure that my environment and food are HEALTHY.
In fact,
I'M AFRAID OF DYING FROM EATING AN UNWASHED TOMATO.
AAAATCHOOO
Murderer!
Or being sneezed on.

There are plenty of other rituals that I have to perform besides medication: mouthwash four times a day, of course, but also blood samples twice per week, to keep an eye on my disease, and changing the dressing on my catheter once per week.

It all takes up a lot of Space

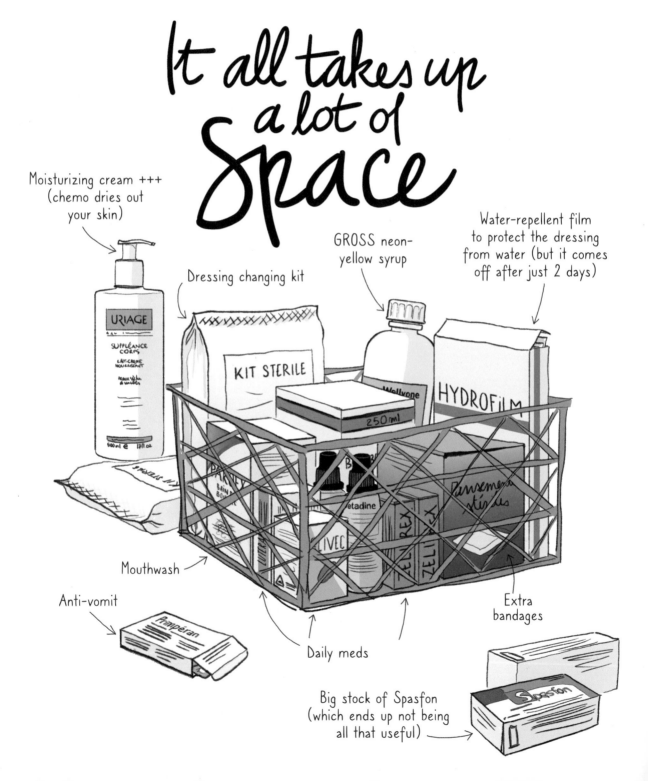

Moisturizing cream +++ (chemo dries out your skin)
Dressing changing kit
GROSS neon-yellow syrup
Water-repellent film to protect the dressing from water (but it comes off after just 2 days)
URIAGE
KIT STERILE
250ml
HYDROFILM
Mouthwash
Anti-vomit
Primpéran
Daily meds
Extra bandages
Big stock of Spasfon (which ends up not being all that useful)
Spasfon

One big difference with the hospital is physical contact. At the hospital, the only moments someone touched me were when the nurse changed my catheter's dressing once a week. Sébastien could hold my hand, but that was it. No kissing, no hugging. I was on my bed and he was in a chair. It seems stupid, but after a month and a half in the hospital, it had gotten really unbearable.

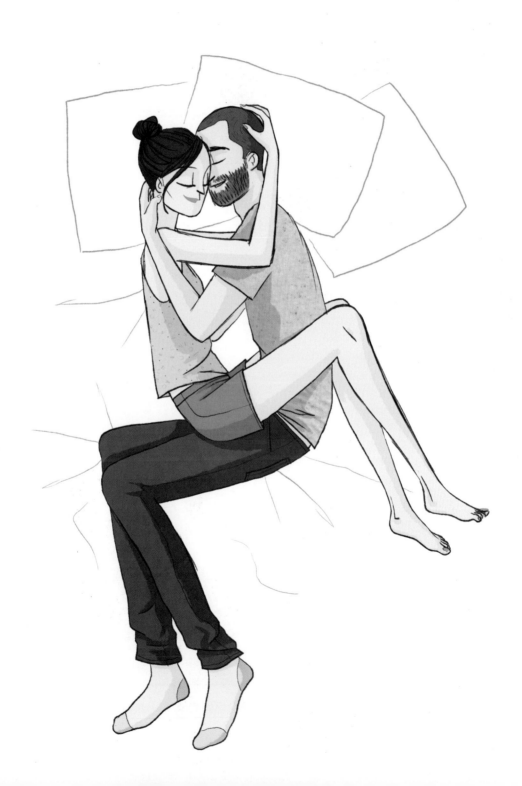

SYMMETRY

Since we're twins, my sister's been worried from the start.

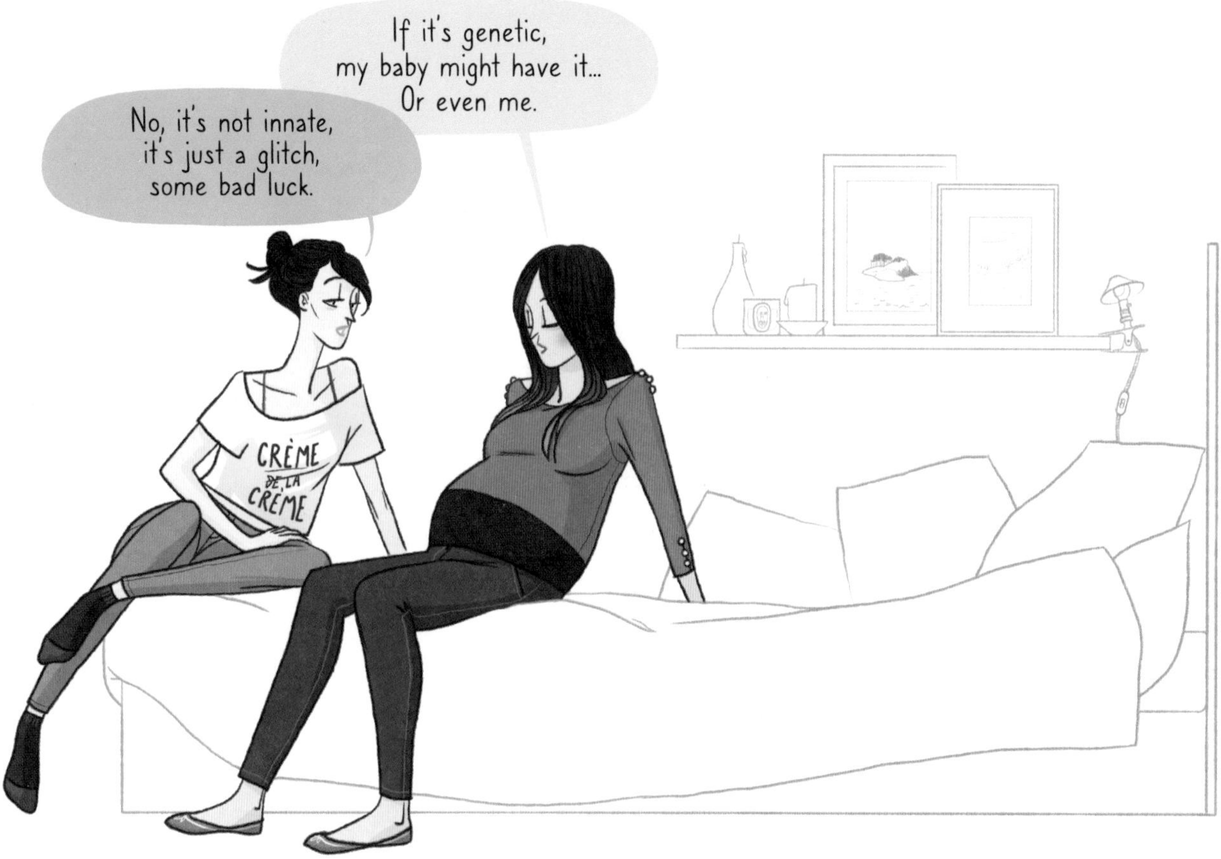
If it's genetic,
my baby might have it...
Or even me.
No, it's not innate,
it's just a glitch,
some bad luck.
CRÈME DE LA CRÈME

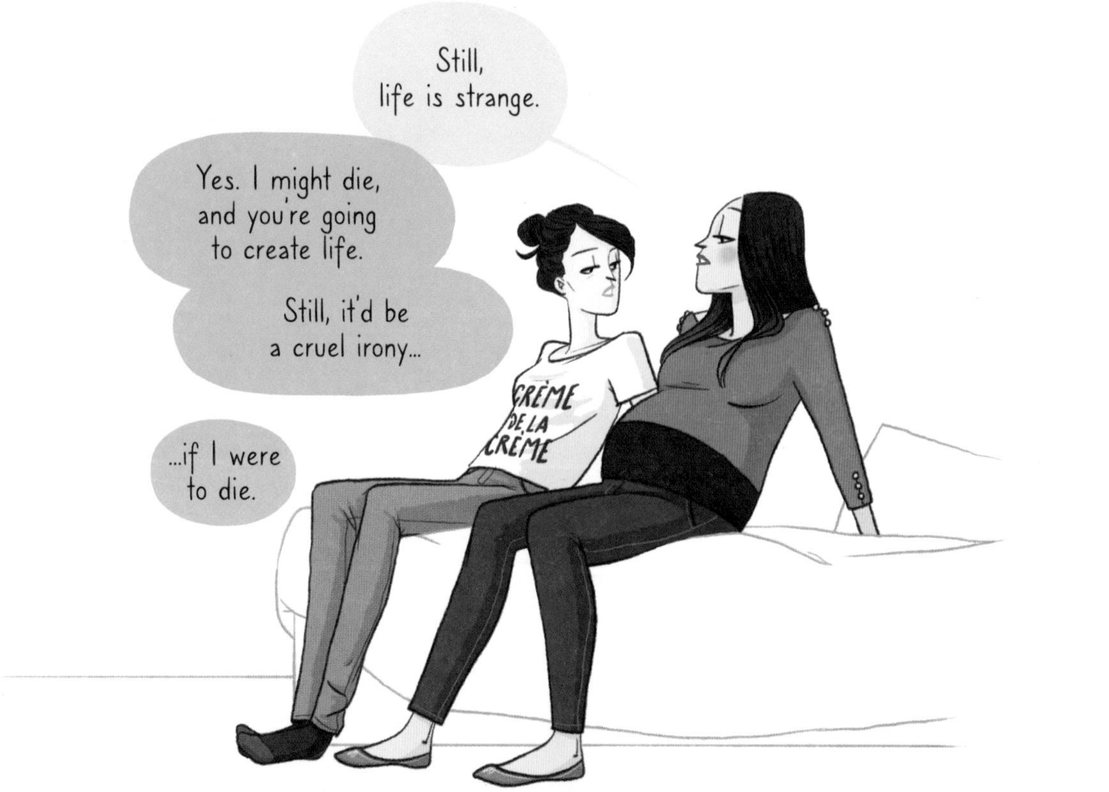
Still,
life is strange.
Yes. I might die,
and you're going
to create life.
Still, it'd be
a cruel irony...
...if I were
to die.
CRÈME DE LA CRÈME

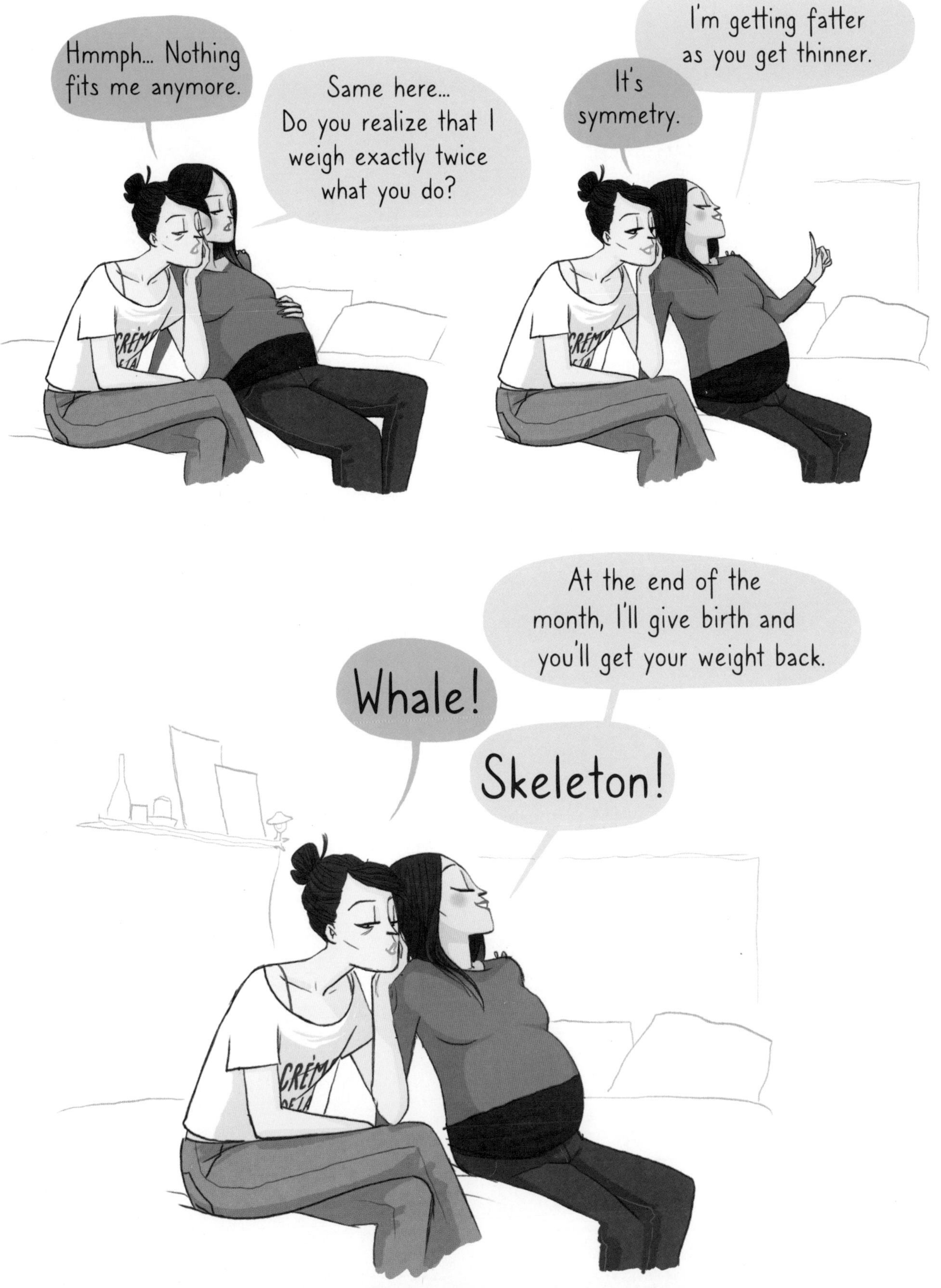
Hmmph... Nothing fits me anymore.
Same here... Do you realize that I weigh exactly twice what you do?
I'm getting fatter as you get thinner.
It's symmetry.
At the end of the month, I'll give birth and you'll get your weight back.
Whale!
Skeleton!

SKELETON

In the tiny mirror in my hospital bathroom, I didn't notice the extent of my weight loss. But once back home, I was in for a big shock...

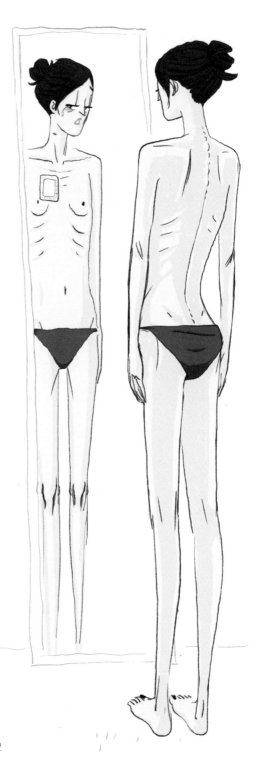

88 pounds. That's scary. It doesn't feel like a "real" number: Aren't you that weight when you're 10? My bones are visible in various places. Vertebrae, sternum, coccyx... I look like I have lines of pebbles under my skin. My withered muscles no longer hide them.

Poor body.

So I've taken things into my own hands. I have about a month to perk up before I go back to the hospital for the first round of chemo. Putting on fat, muscle, **GO GIRL!**

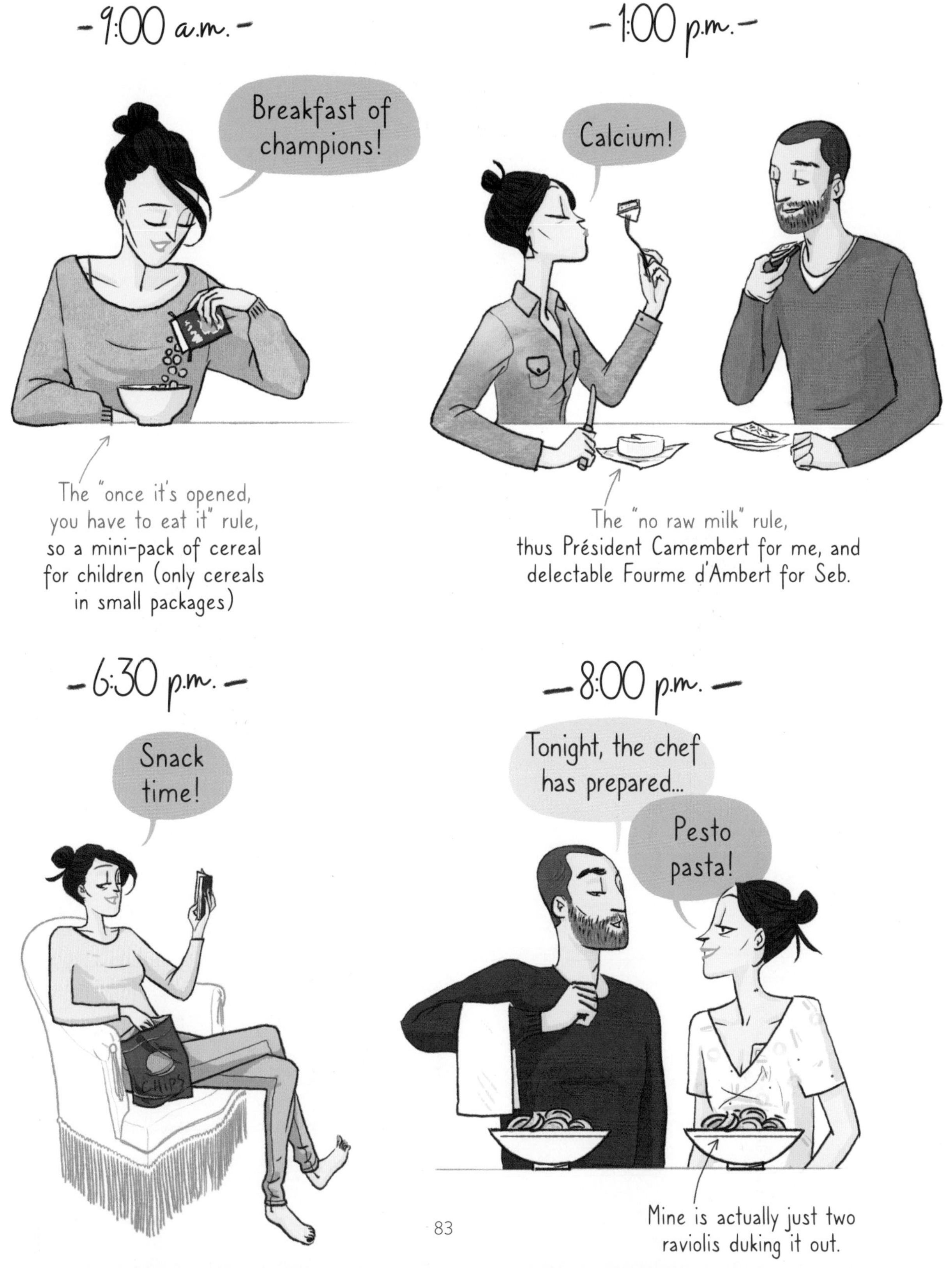
-9:00 a.m.-
Breakfast of champions!
The "once it's opened, you have to eat it" rule, so a mini-pack of cereal for children (only cereals in small packages)
-1:00 p.m.-
Calcium!
The "no raw milk" rule, thus Président Camembert for me, and delectable Fourme d'Ambert for Seb.
-6:30 p.m.-
Snack time!
CHIPS
-8:00 p.m.-
Tonight, the chef has prepared...
Pesto pasta!
Mine is actually just two raviolis duking it out.

I'M SHEDDING ALL OVER THE PLACE

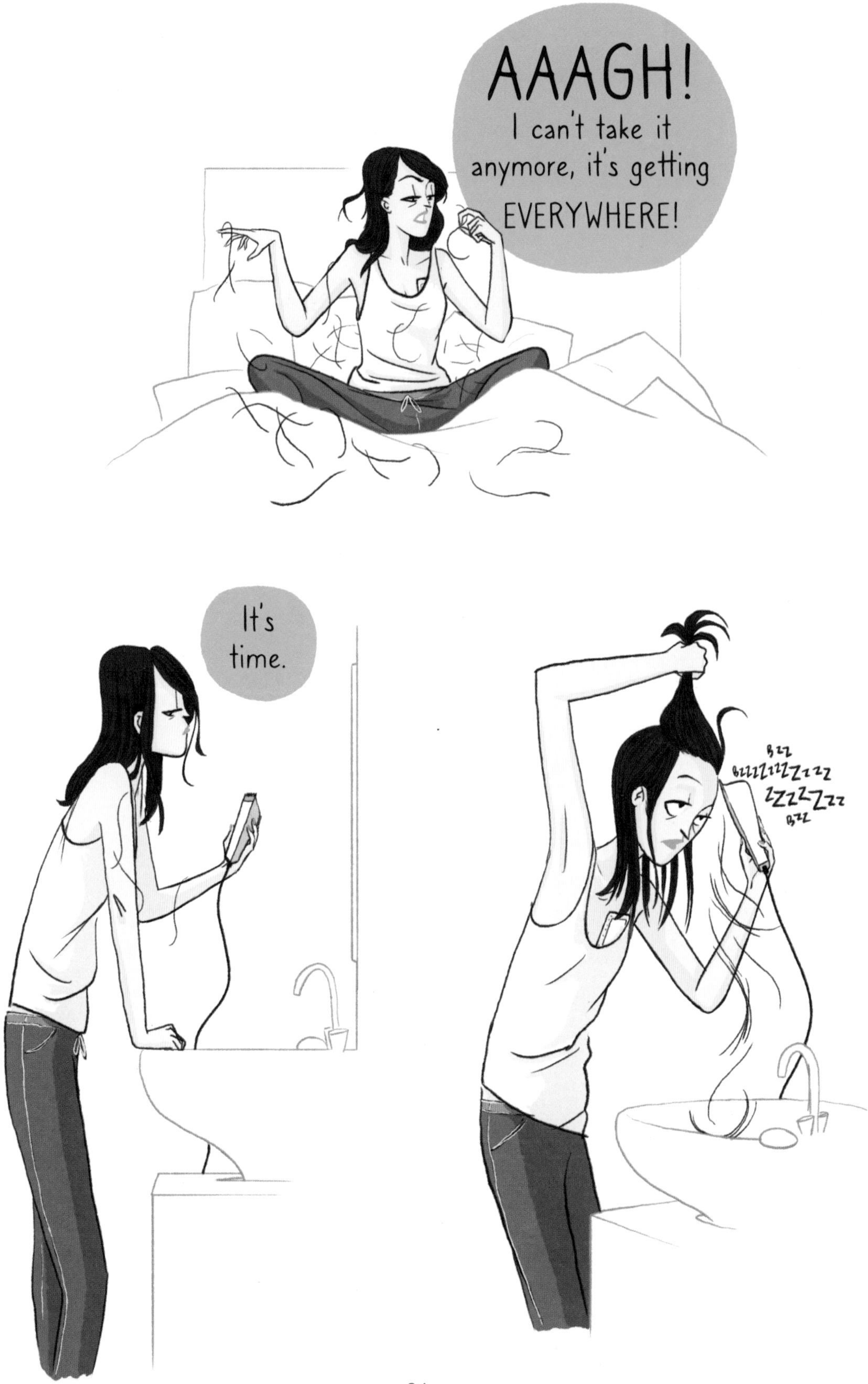
AAAGH!
I can't take it anymore, it's getting EVERYWHERE!
It's time.
BZZ
BZZZZZZZZZZZZ
ZZZZZZzz
BZZ

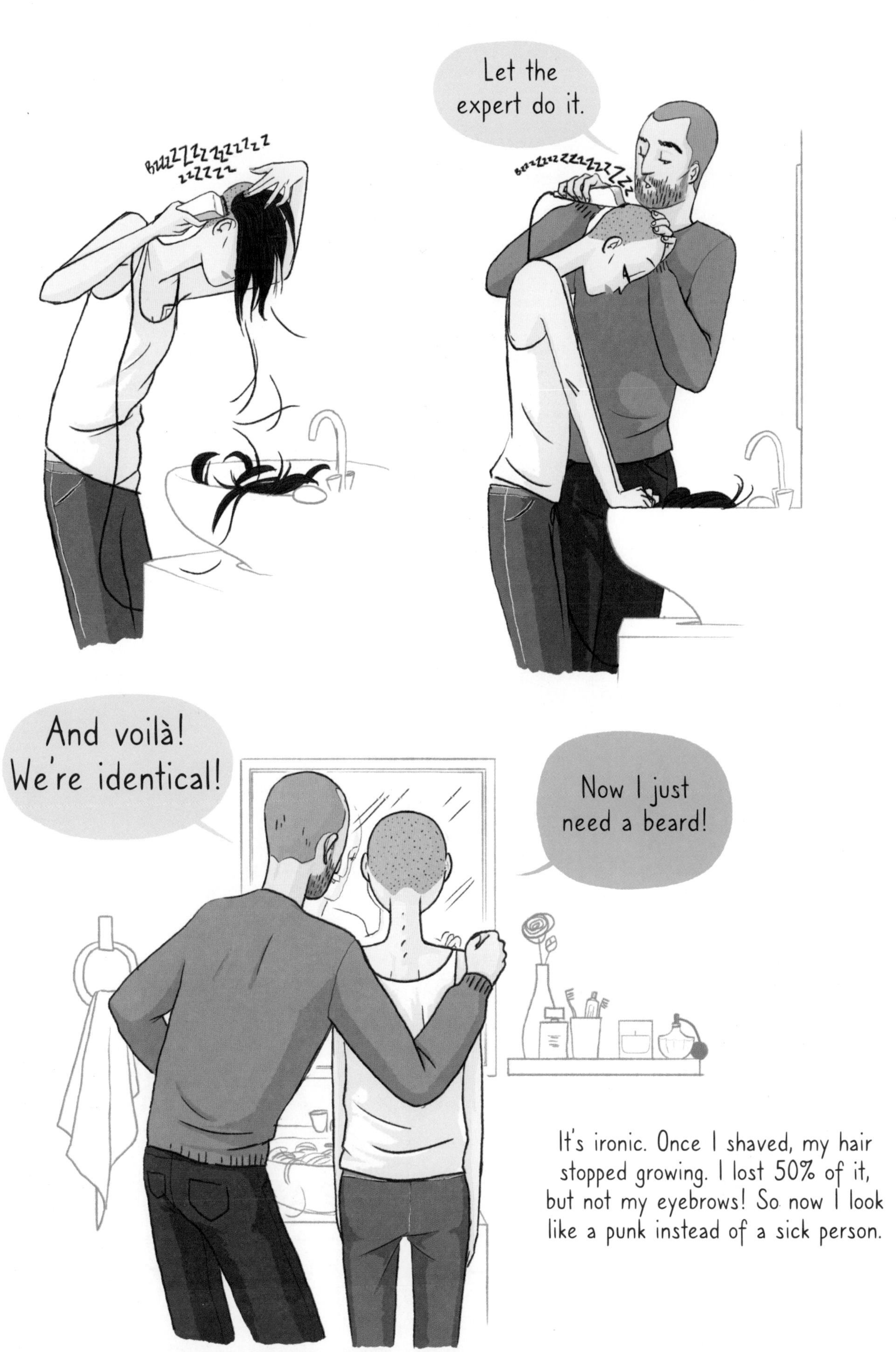
Let the expert do it.
And voilà! We're identical!
Now I just need a beard!
It's ironic. Once I shaved, my hair stopped growing. I lost 50% of it, but not my eyebrows! So now I look like a punk instead of a sick person.

THE GAZE OF OTHERS

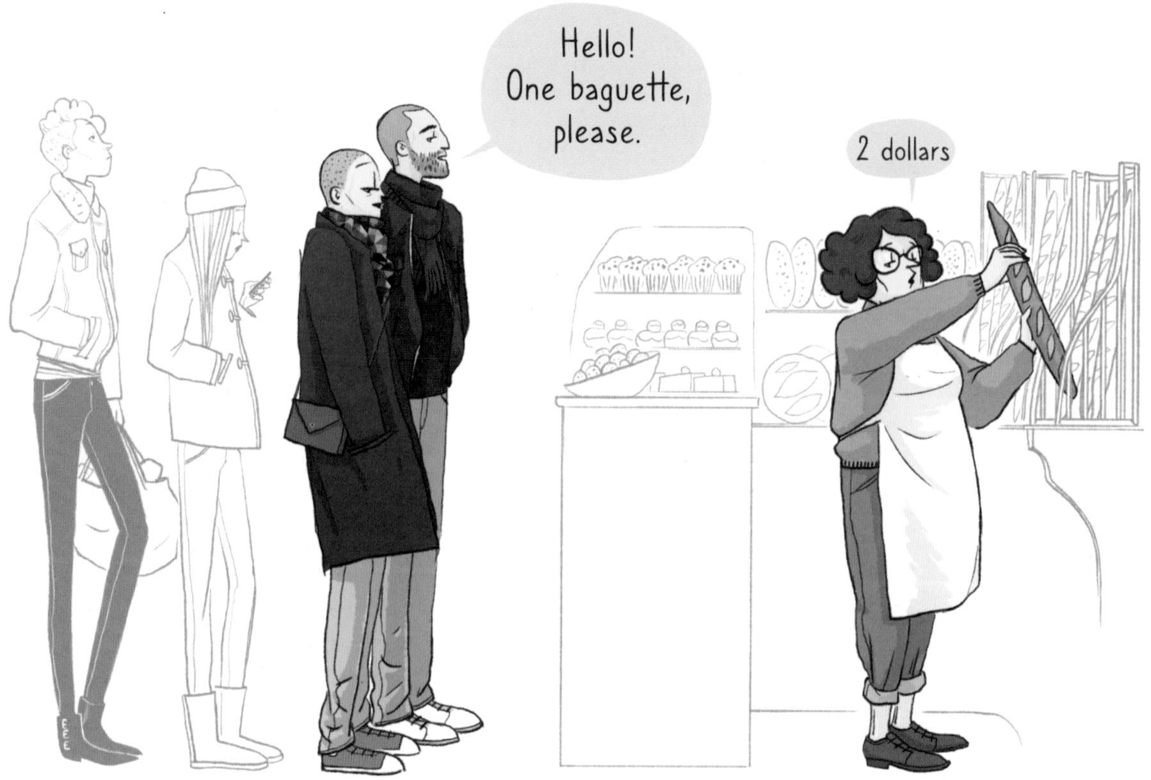
Hello! One baguette, please.
2 dollars

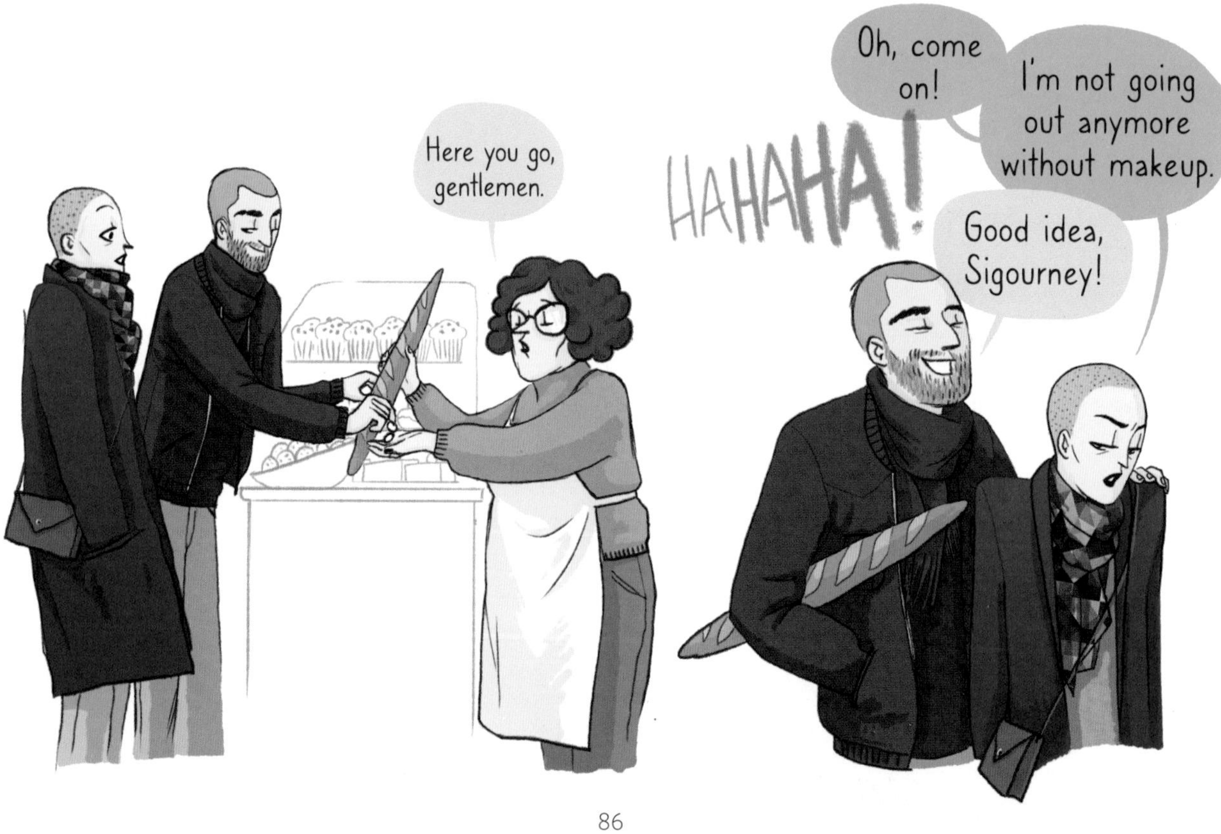
Here you go, gentlemen.
HAHAHA!
Oh, come on!
I'm not going out anymore without makeup.
Good idea, Sigourney!

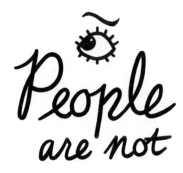

People are not

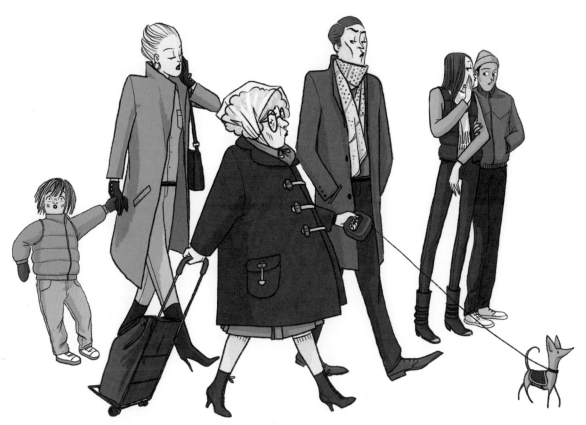

very discreet

The older ones often give me a side glance, while
the younger ones stare with their mouths open.

A NEW ROUTINE

This "out of the hospital" period is like a vacation. A digression, a bubble. 2015 doesn't count; it'll be a year apart. No work, no hair, but in good hands.

MORNING

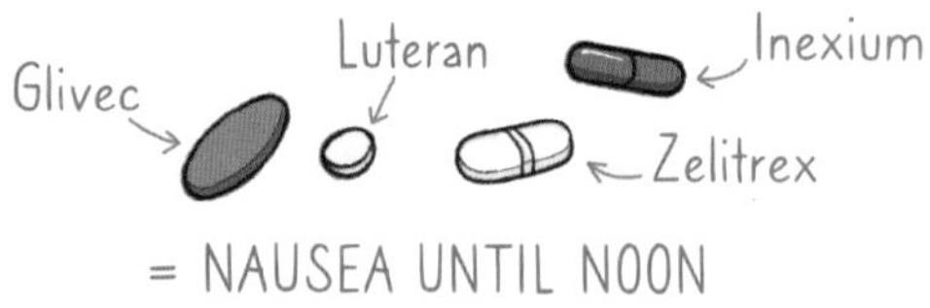
Glivec
Luteran
Inexium
Zelitrex
= NAUSEA UNTIL NOON

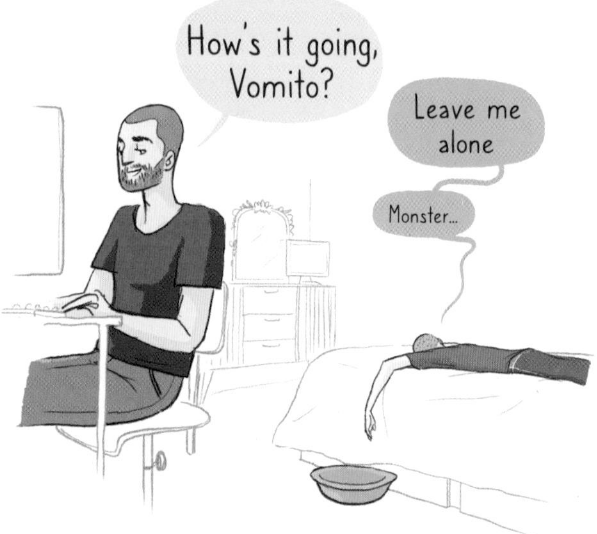
How's it going, Vomito?
Leave me alone
Monster...

NOON

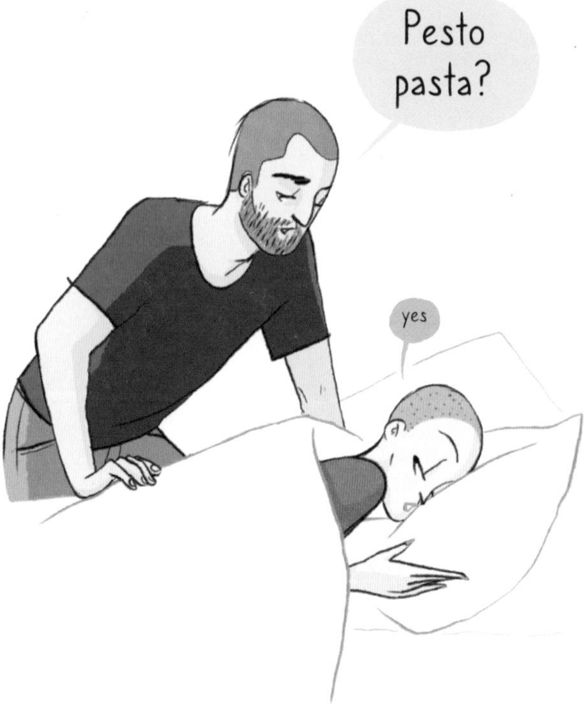
Pesto pasta?
yes

AFTERNOON

Ritual stroll, every day a little farther, with my "SUPER SHOPPING ALIBI"—or, as my sister calls it, my "LEUKEMIA CARD."

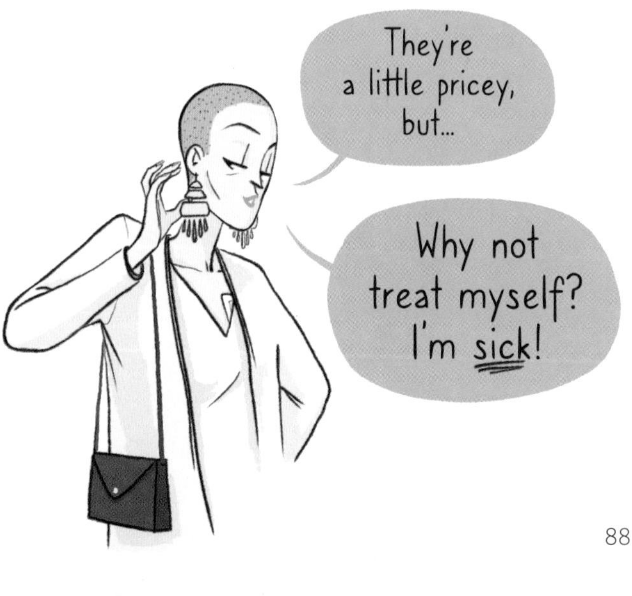
They're a little pricey, but...
Why not treat myself? I'm sick!

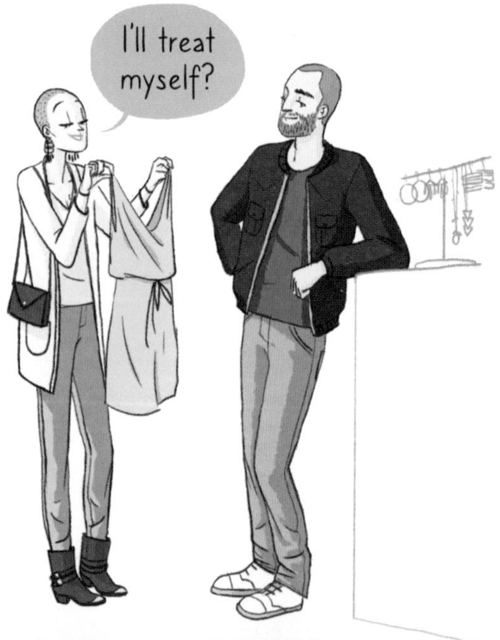
I'll treat myself?

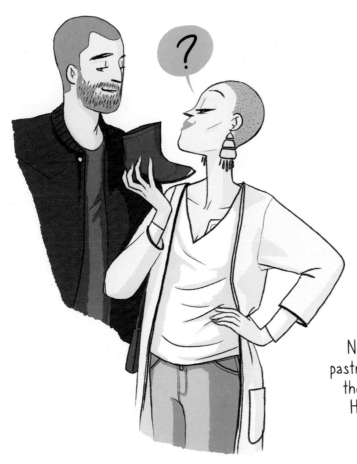

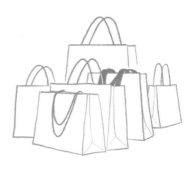

My LEUKEMIA CARD also works
on plenty of other things.
—
Not doing the dishes, eating the last
pastry, buying myself a drink, not carrying
the groceries, deciding on dinner, etc.
However, I can't overdo it if I want
to keep the "scam" going.

EVENING

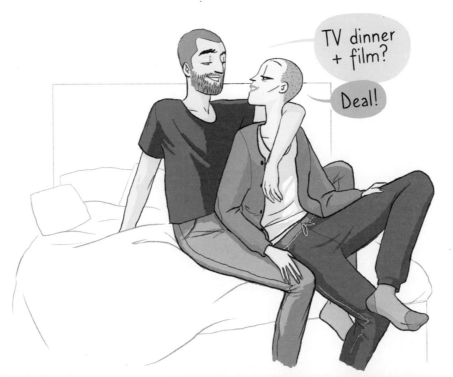

GLASS HALF FULL

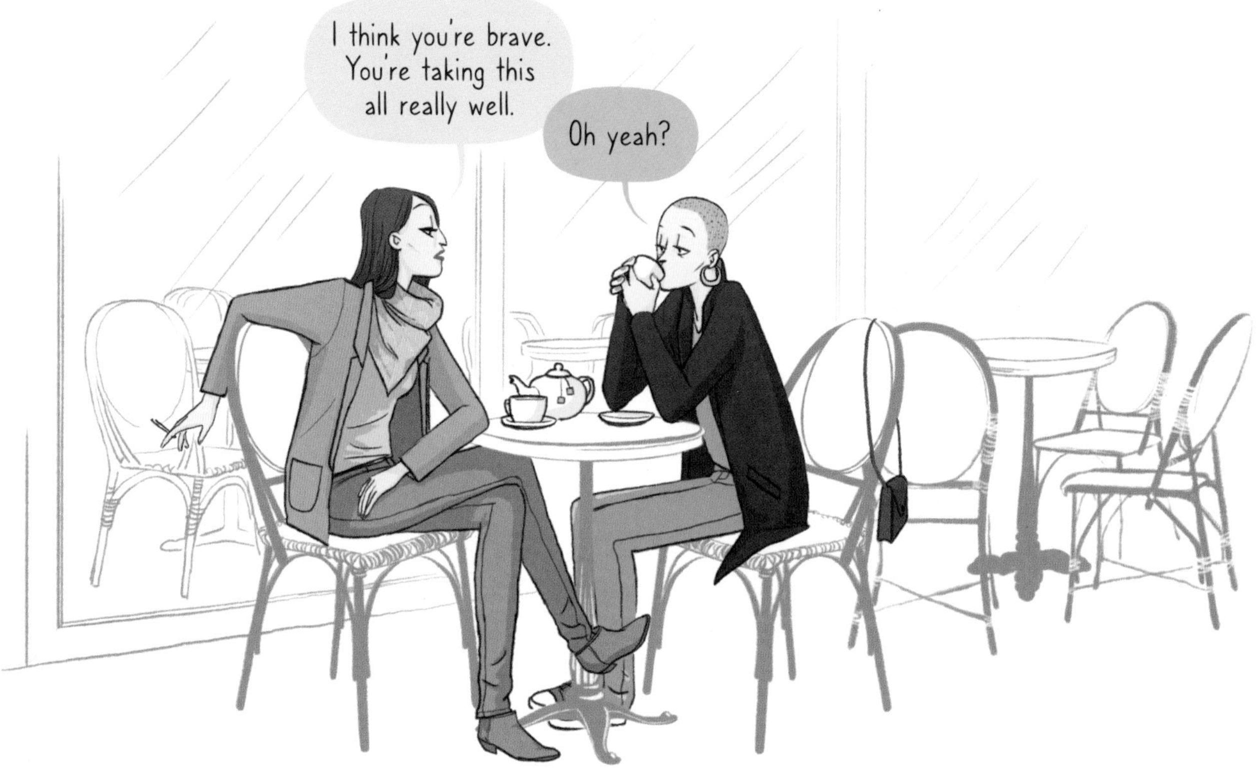
I think you're brave. You're taking this all really well.
Oh yeah?

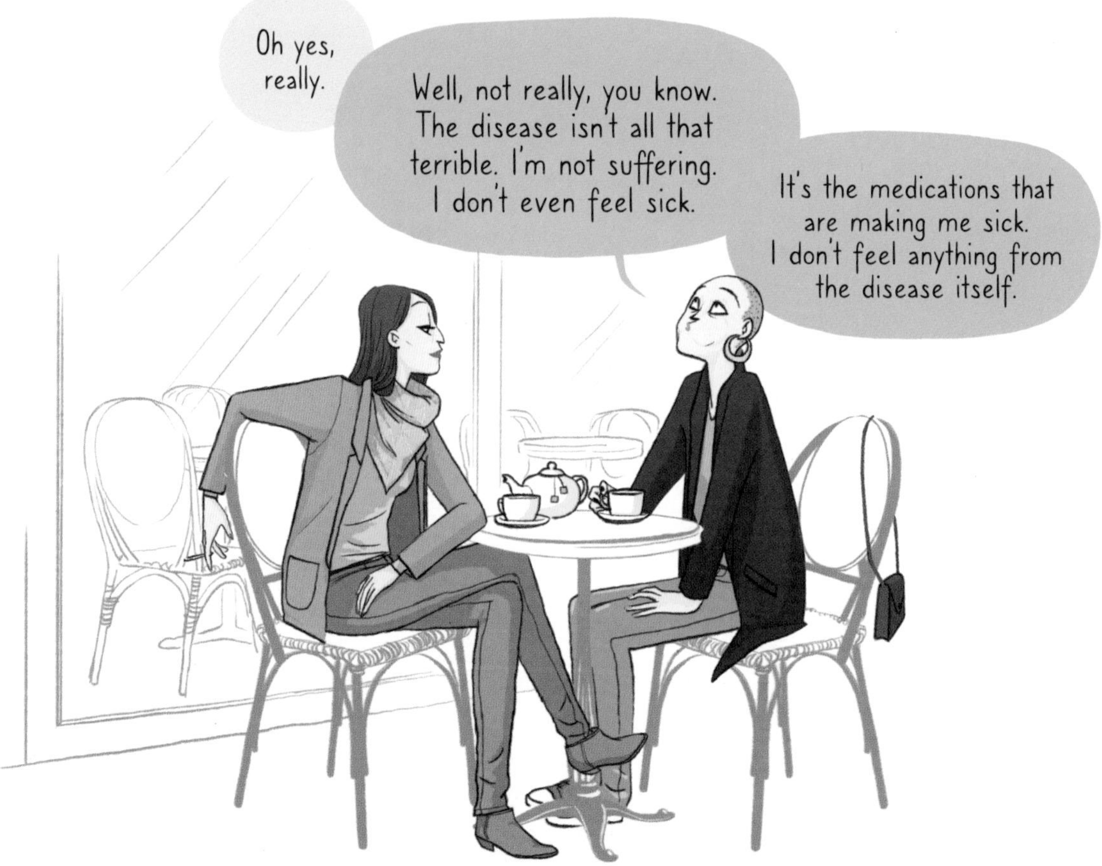
Oh yes, really.
Well, not really, you know. The disease isn't all that terrible. I'm not suffering. I don't even feel sick.
It's the medications that are making me sick. I don't feel anything from the disease itself.

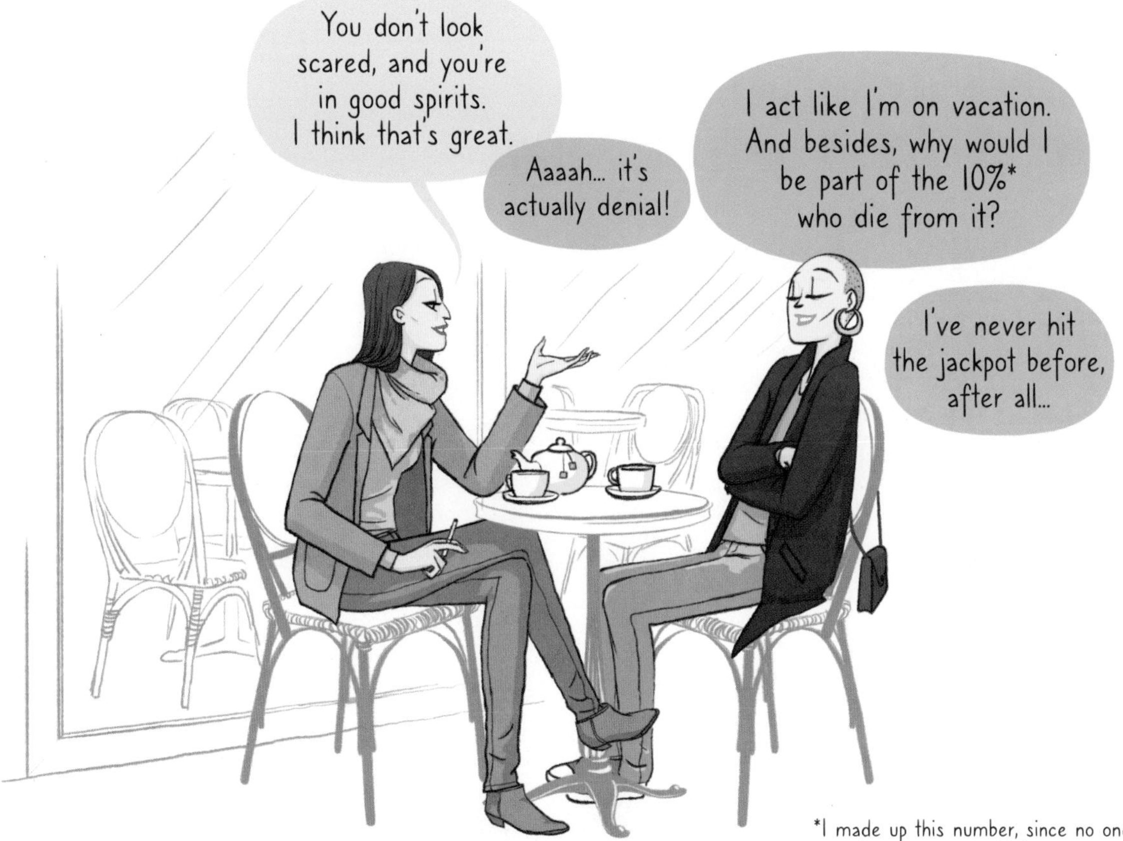
You don't look scared, and you're in good spirits. I think that's great.
Aaaah... it's actually denial!
I act like I'm on vacation. And besides, why would I be part of the 10%* who die from it?
I've never hit the jackpot before, after all...

*I made up this number, since no one wanted to tell me the truth. 10% is fine, not too scary.

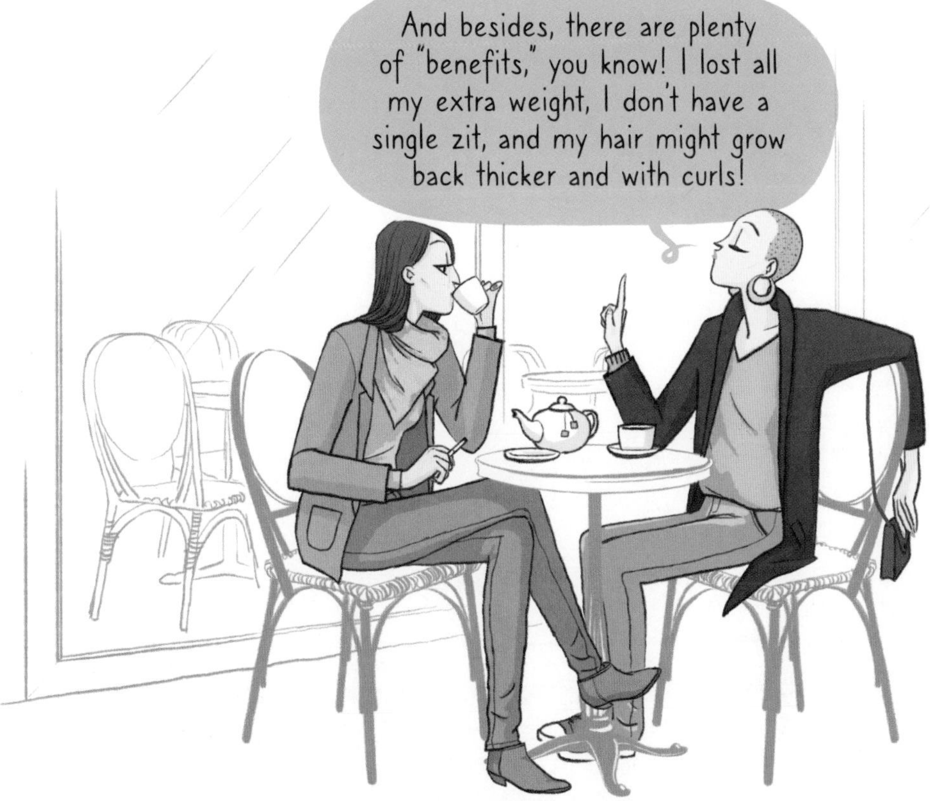
And besides, there are plenty of "benefits," you know! I lost all my extra weight, I don't have a single zit, and my hair might grow back thicker and with curls!

MY COST OF LIVING

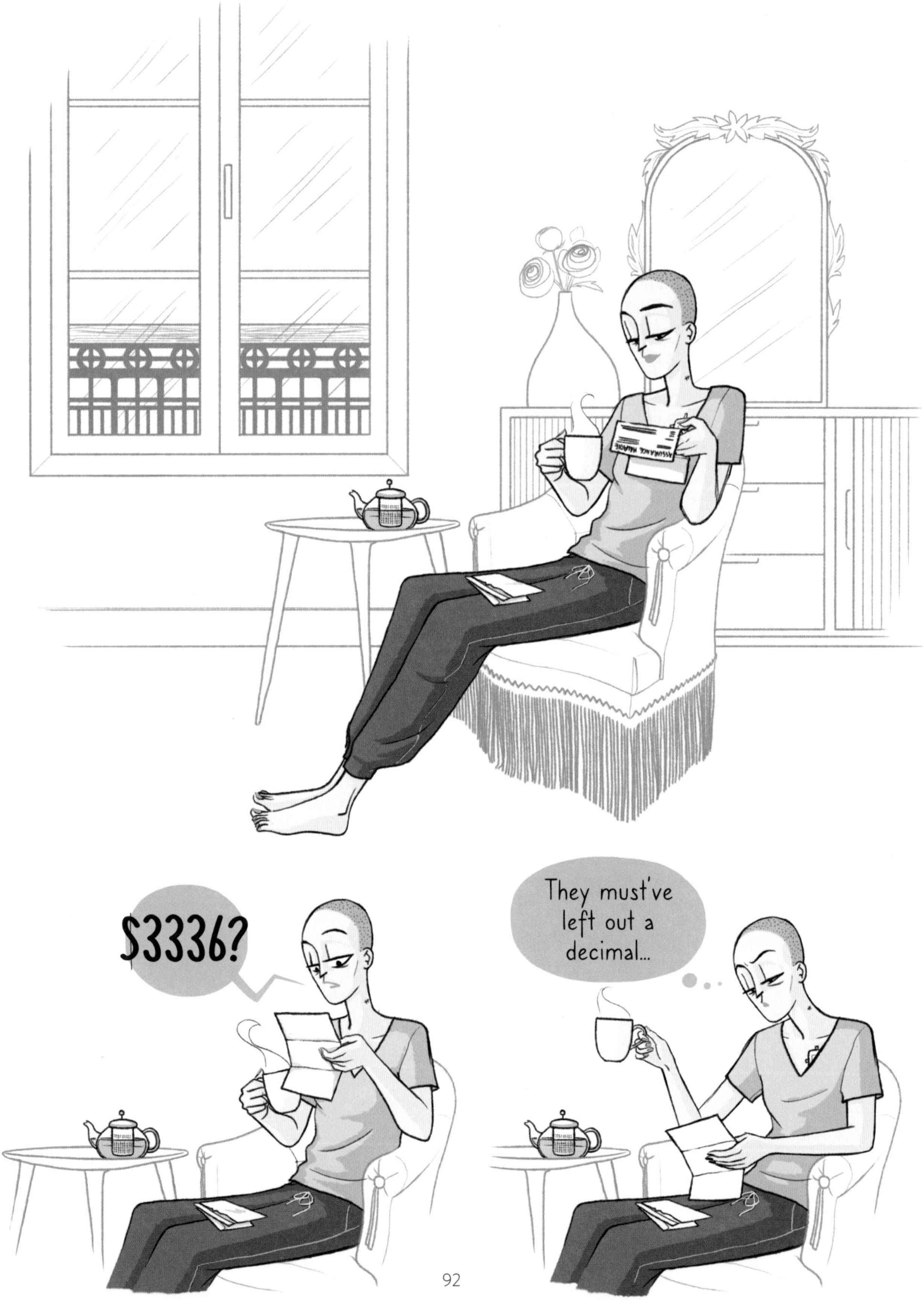
$3336?
They must've left out a decimal...

Everything leukemia-related is taken care of 100% by Social Security. I don't pay a dime, but I still get statements for my pharmacy costs.

There's no way one month of meds costs that much!

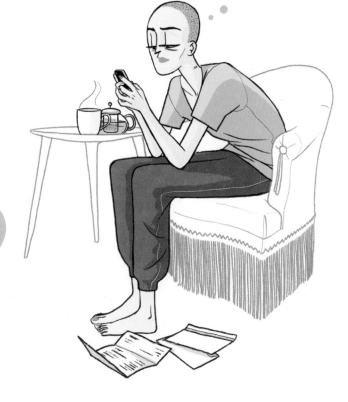

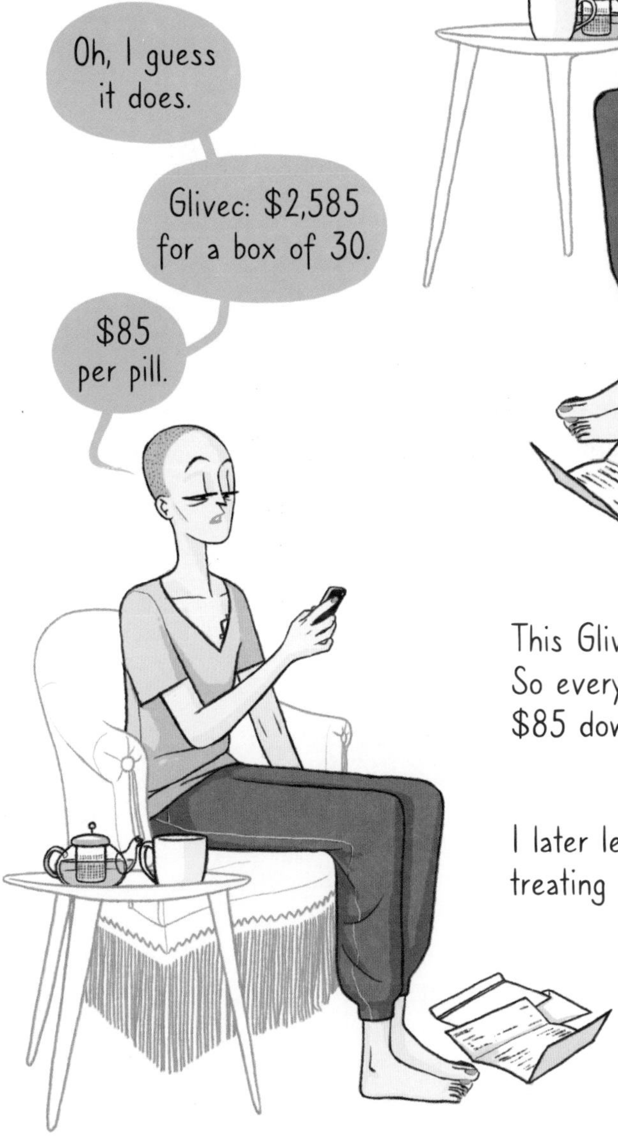

Oh, I guess it does.

Glivec: $2,585 for a box of 30.

$85 per pill.

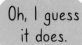

This Glivec medication makes me really nauseated. So every time I throw up, I'm flushing at least $85 down the drain.

I later learned that the average cost for treating leukemia is $274,000.

PUTTING MY EGGS IN A NEW BASKET

I have an appointment at the Poissy-St Germain Hospital with Dr. Poirot, a fertility specialist, since the doctors told me that the transplant chemo (in June) might leave me sterile.

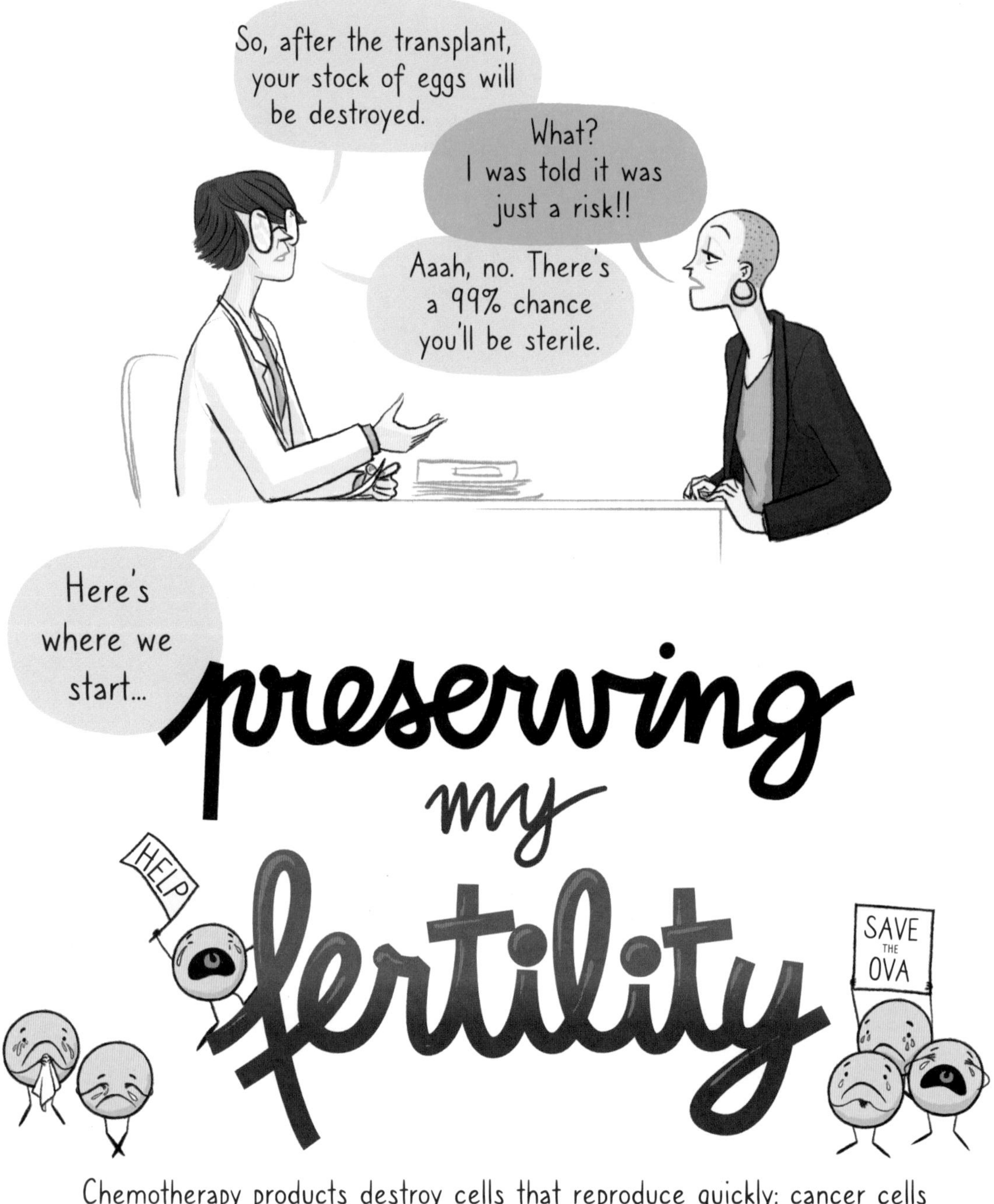
So, after the transplant, your stock of eggs will be destroyed.
What? I was told it was just a risk!!
Aaah, no. There's a 99% chance you'll be sterile.
Here's where we start...
preserving my fertility
HELP
SAVE THE OVA

Chemotherapy products destroy cells that reproduce quickly: cancer cells but also **HEAD HAIR** (as in my case, though not completely), **BODY HAIR** (a little for me, but thankfully not my eyebrows!), and sometimes even **NAILS!** (Not in my case, phew! It depends on the products used.) Before the transplant, I'll have one last chemo to burn allll the cancer cells still left in my bone marrow, but that chemo will also destroy **MY OVA...**

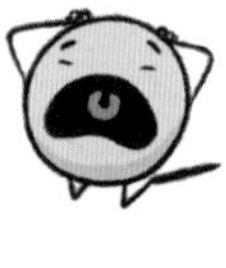

AND THERE'S THE PROBLEM!

Men can produce sperm cells their entire lives, but for women, all future ova are formed **BEFORE** birth. Then, throughout adolescence, one ovarian follicle matures each month. But the stock doesn't grow back; it's exhausted little by little. So after the pre-transplant chemo, my whole stock will be **DESTROYED!**

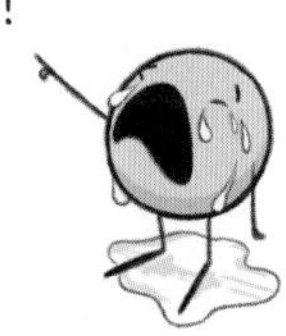

SO WHAT DO WE DO?

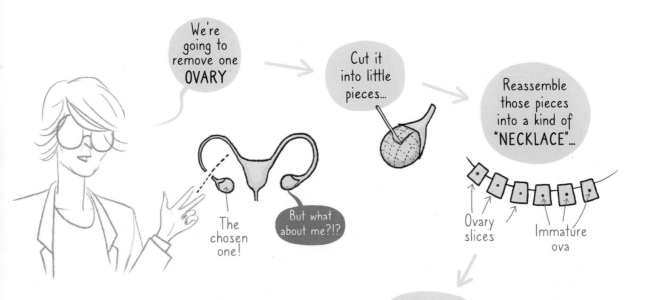

We're going to remove one **OVARY**

The chosen one!

But what about me?!?

Cut it into little pieces...

Reassemble those pieces into a kind of **"NECKLACE"**...

Ovary slices

Immature ova

And freeze the whole thing!

Once I decide to have a child, this "necklace" will be implanted back inside me,

AND HERE'S THE MAGIC PART... 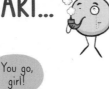 BUT!!!

The little ovary bits will start working again on their own, acting like an ovary, and thus one ovum a month, **AS IF NOTHING HAD HAPPENED!**

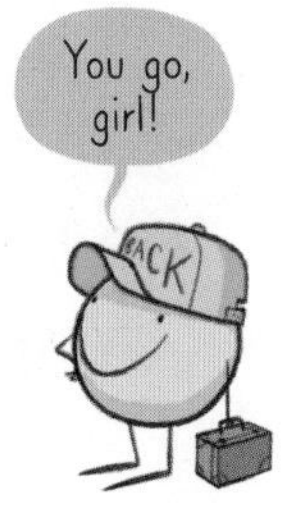

You go, girl!

THERE'S A CHANCE IT WON'T WORK:
-the freezing could fail,
-the leukemia might be present in the sample (in that case, doctor's veto, she won't reimplant them).

My next appointment is at the Pitié-Salpêtrière Hospital with Dr. Fortin, the surgeon who's going to remove my ovary.

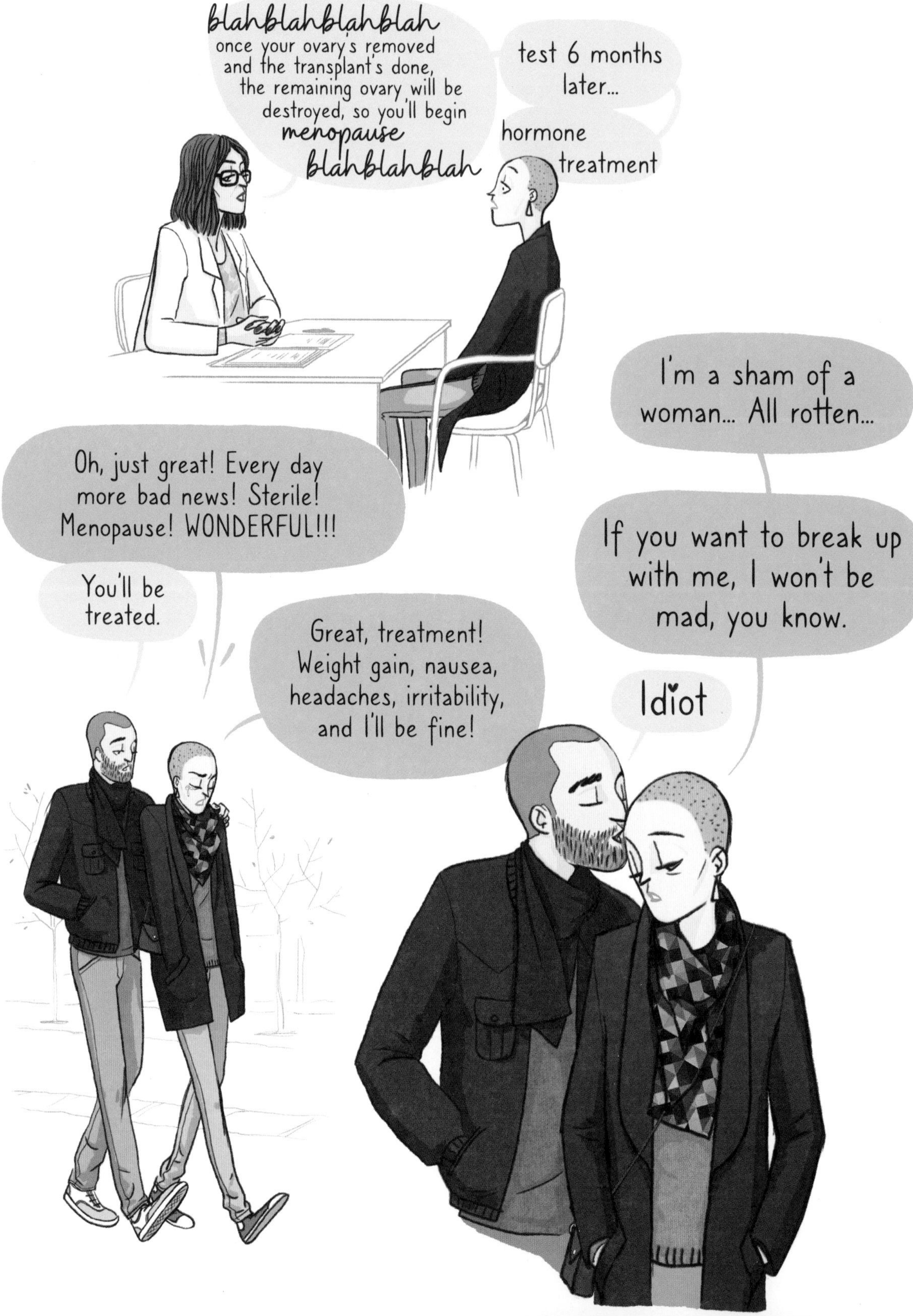
blahblahblahblah once your ovary's removed and the transplant's done, the remaining ovary will be destroyed, so you'll begin menopause blahblahblah
test 6 months later...
hormone treatment
Oh, just great! Every day more bad news! Sterile! Menopause! WONDERFUL!!!
You'll be treated.
Great, treatment! Weight gain, nausea, headaches, irritability, and I'll be fine!
I'm a sham of a woman... All rotten...
If you want to break up with me, I won't be mad, you know.
Idiot

GENETICS

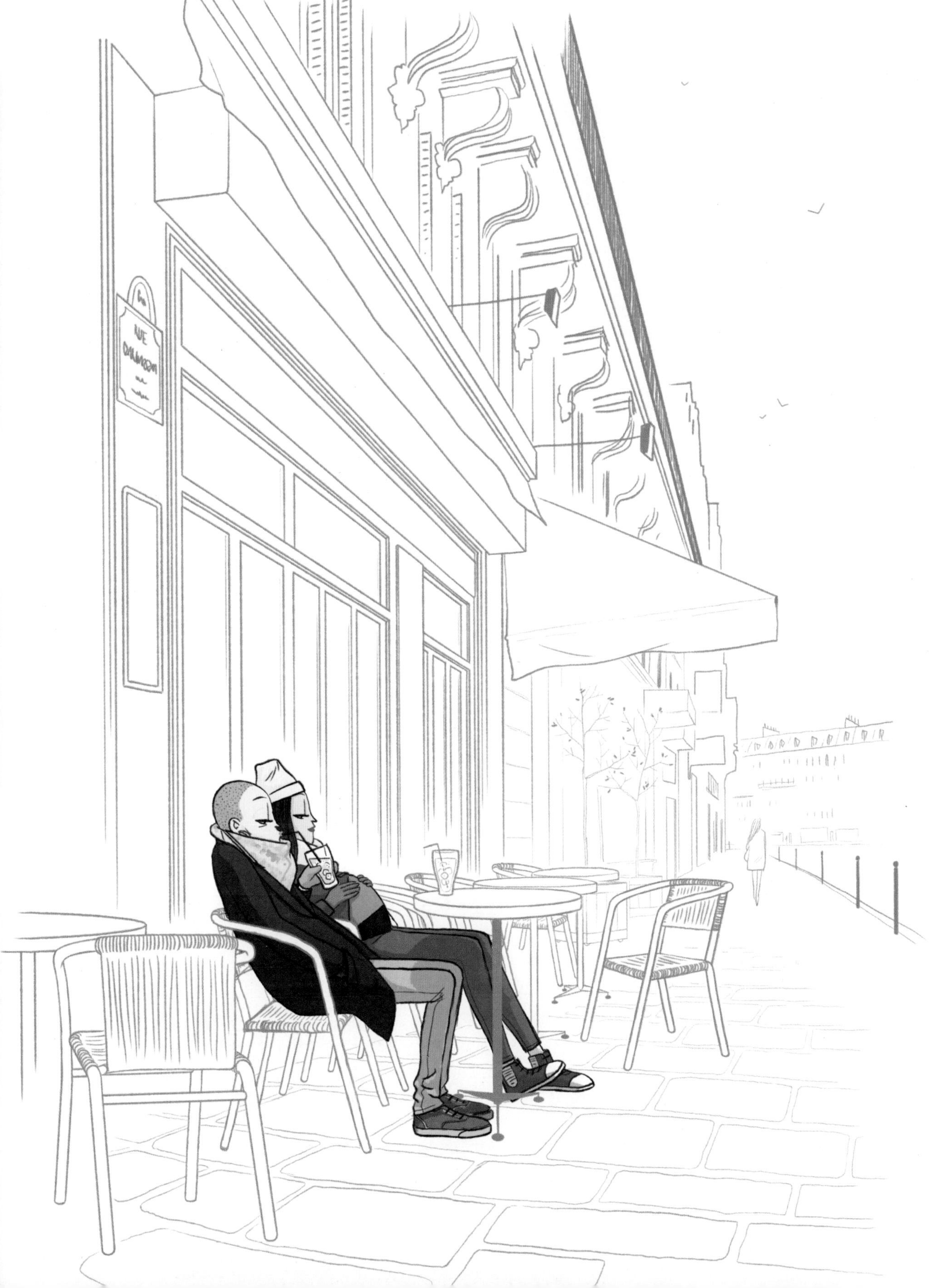

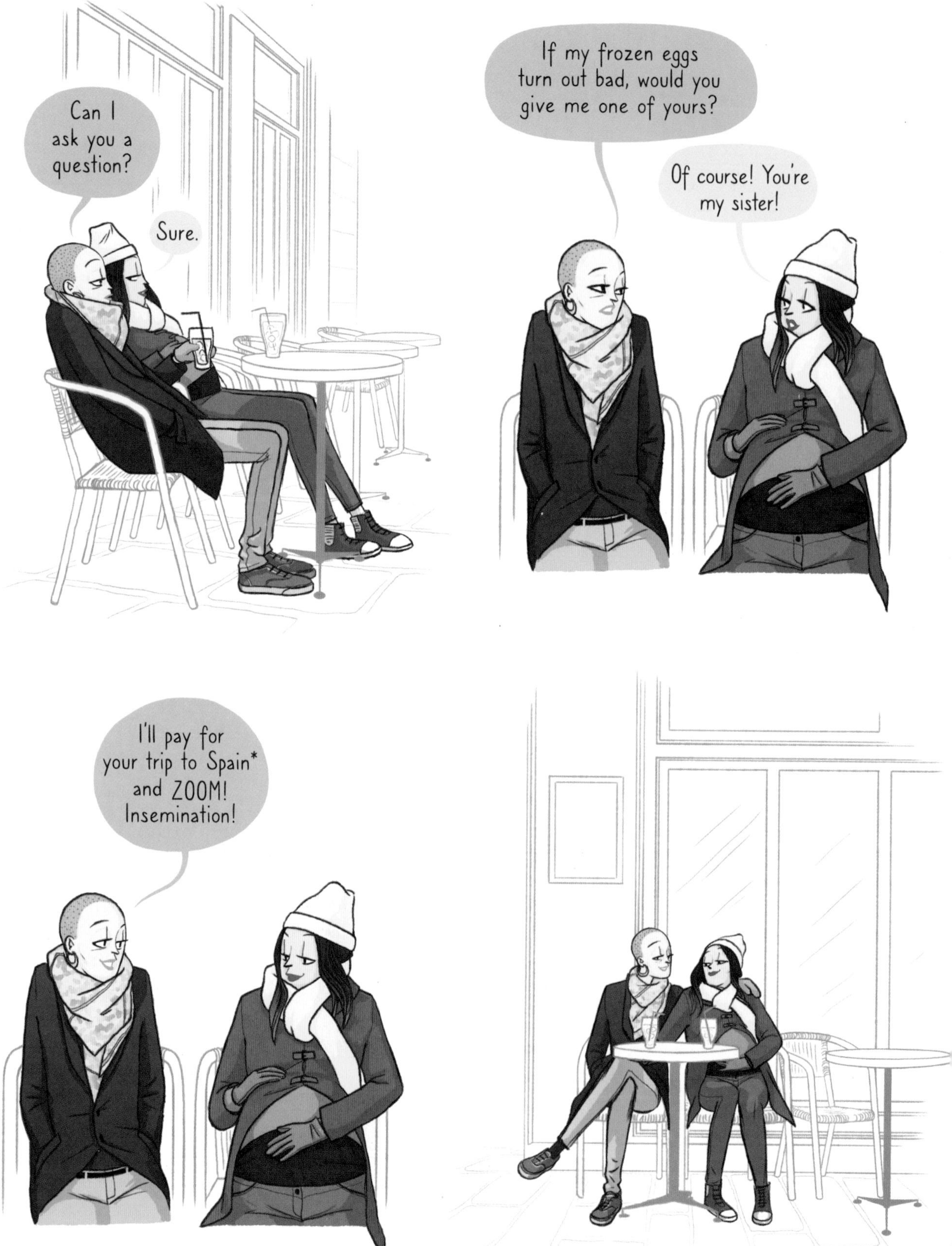
Can I ask you a question?
Sure.
If my frozen eggs turn out bad, would you give me one of yours?
Of course! You're my sister!
I'll pay for your trip to Spain* and ZOOM! Insemination!

*In France, oocyte donation is anonymous, so you can't decide who receives your gift.

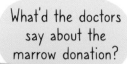

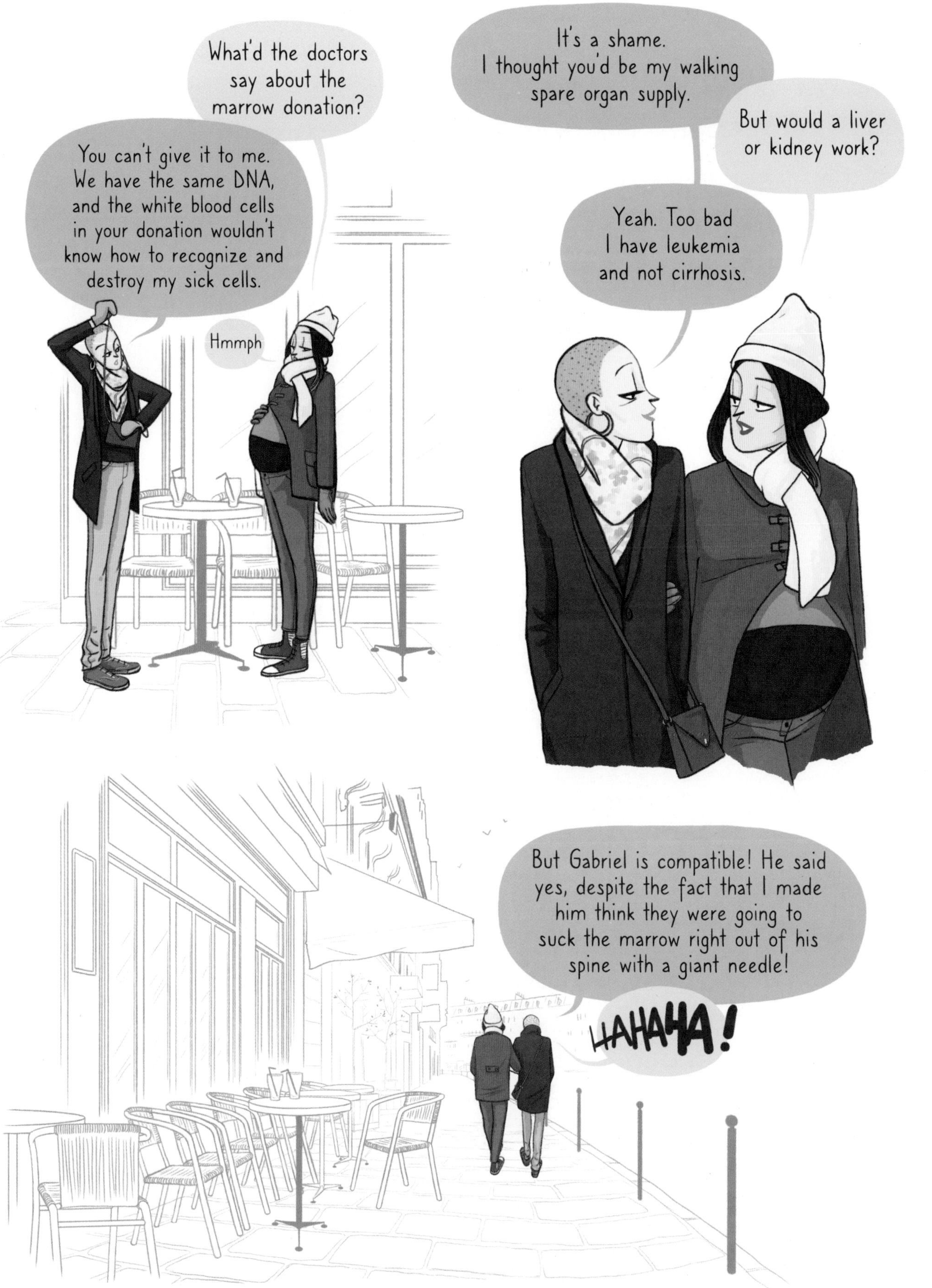

What'd the doctors say about the marrow donation?

It's a shame. I thought you'd be my walking spare organ supply.

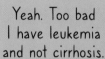

But would a liver or kidney work?

You can't give it to me. We have the same DNA, and the white blood cells in your donation wouldn't know how to recognize and destroy my sick cells.

Yeah. Too bad I have leukemia and not cirrhosis.

Hmmph

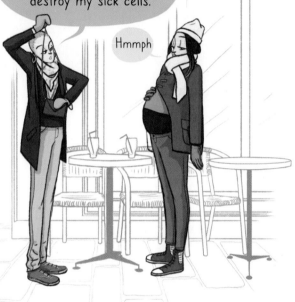

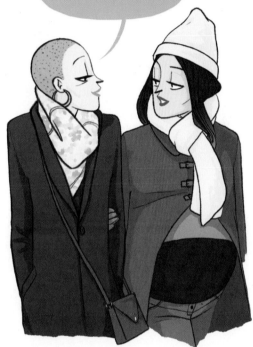

But Gabriel is compatible! He said yes, despite the fact that I made him think they were going to suck the marrow right out of his spine with a giant needle!

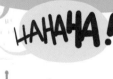

HAHAHA!

THE GANG OF BALDIES

At the end of January, my sister gave birth to magnificent little Daphné.

BOOM!
Check out this masterpiece!

Heh, hey you!

She's been born, and I'm not dead. I'm sure that everything will be fine!

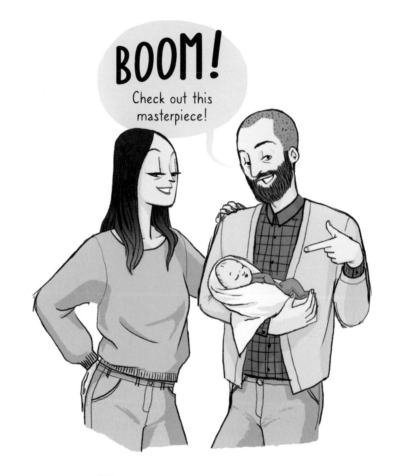

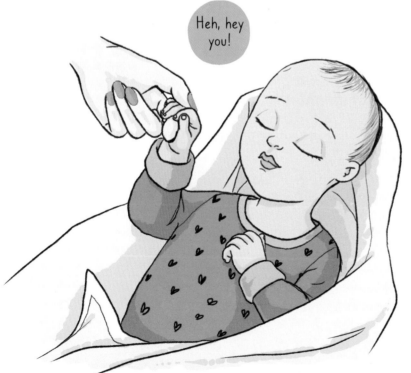

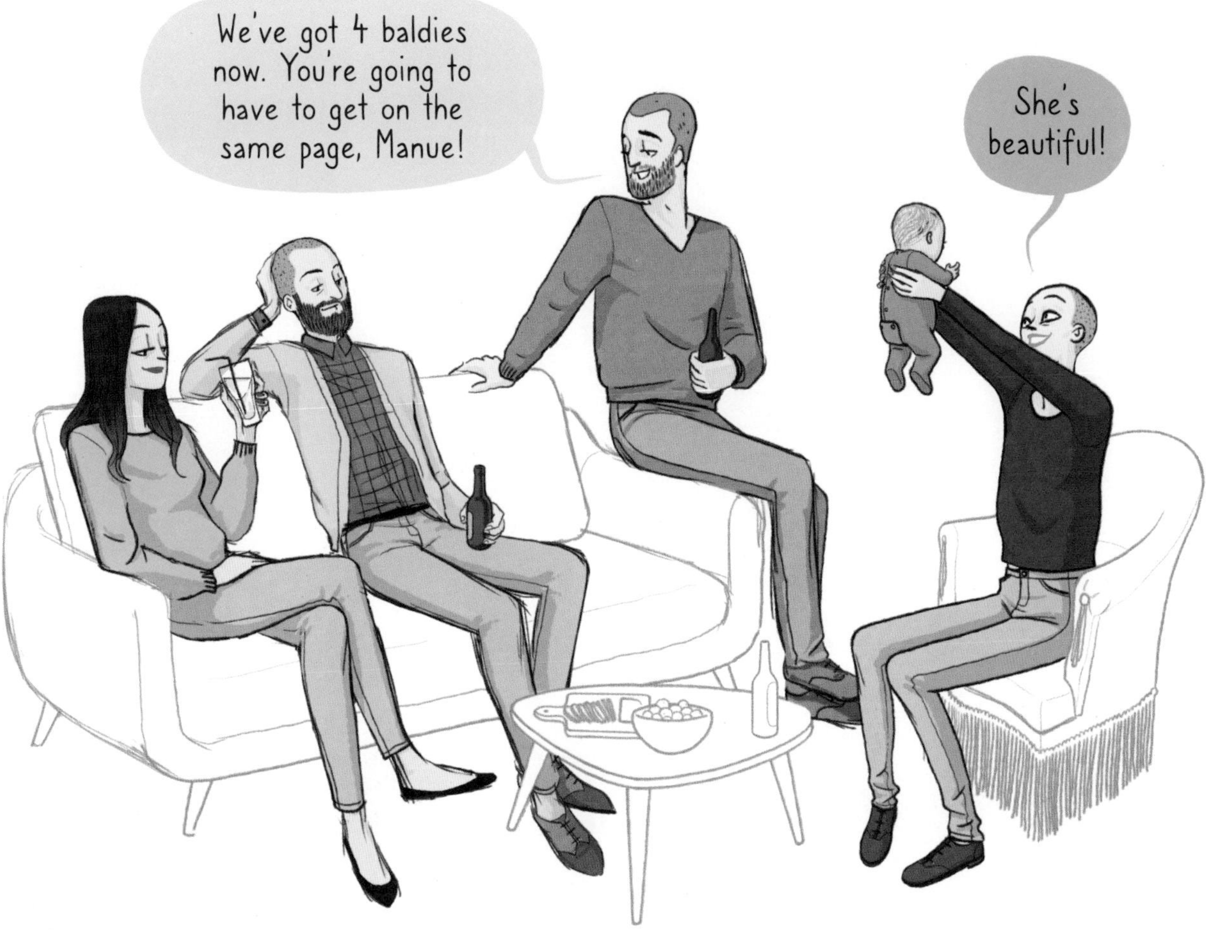
We've got 4 baldies now. You're going to have to get on the same page, Manue!
She's beautiful!

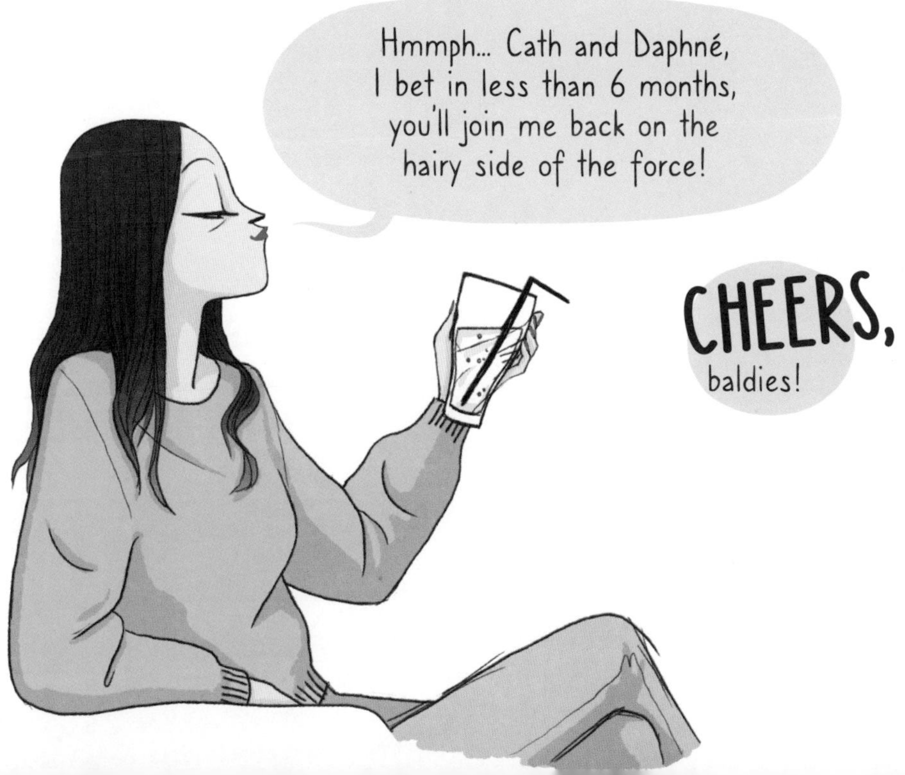
Hmmph... Cath and Daphné, I bet in less than 6 months, you'll join me back on the hairy side of the force!
CHEERS, baldies!

FEBRUARY 12

DONE QUICK, DONE RIGHT

Return to the hospital for the **FIRST ROUND OF CONSOLIDATION CHEMO**. The goal of this treatment is to prevent any new growth of cancer cells while the patient is in remission (temporary remission, since without a bone marrow transplant I'll end up relapsing). Time to consolidate!

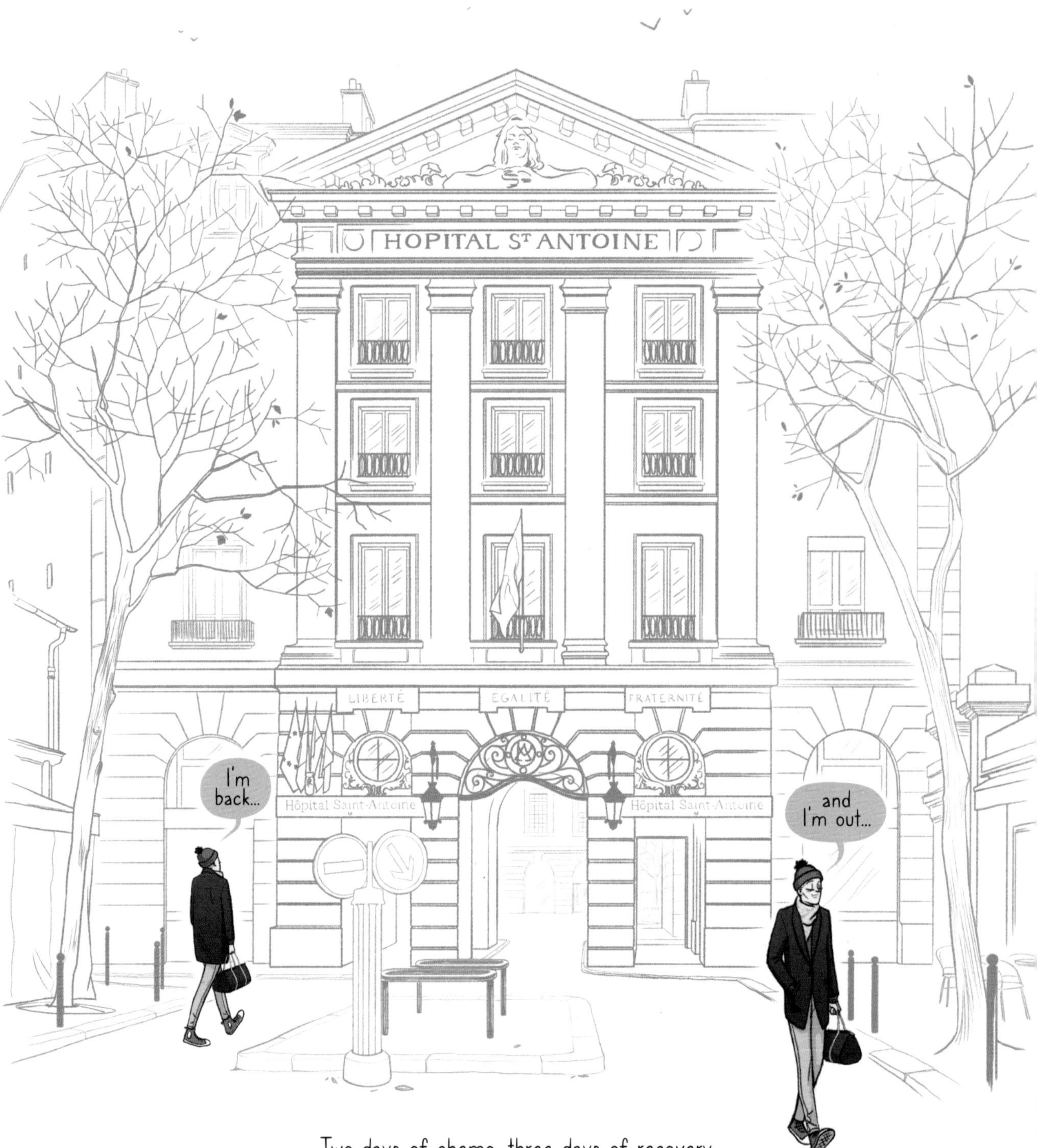
HOPITAL St ANTOINE
LIBERTÉ
EGALITÉ
FRATERNITÉ
Hôpital Saint-Antoine
Hôpital Saint-Antoine
I'm back...
and I'm out...

Two days of chemo, three days of recovery, and BOOM! I'm out! See you next month.

OPERATION SCRAMBLED EGGS

March 3—At the hospital for the removal of my ovary. It's my first operation, and I'm a little apprehensive...

SHOWER

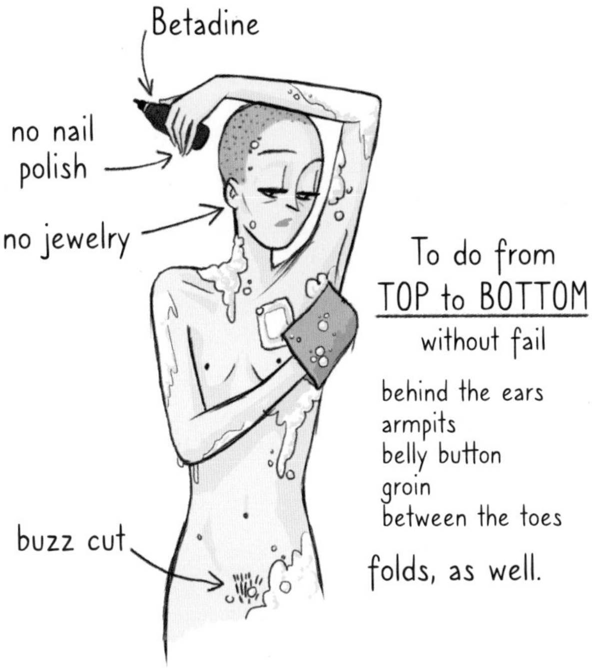

Betadine
no nail polish
no jewelry
buzz cut
To do from TOP to BOTTOM without fail
behind the ears
armpits
belly button
groin
between the toes
folds, as well.

OUTFIT

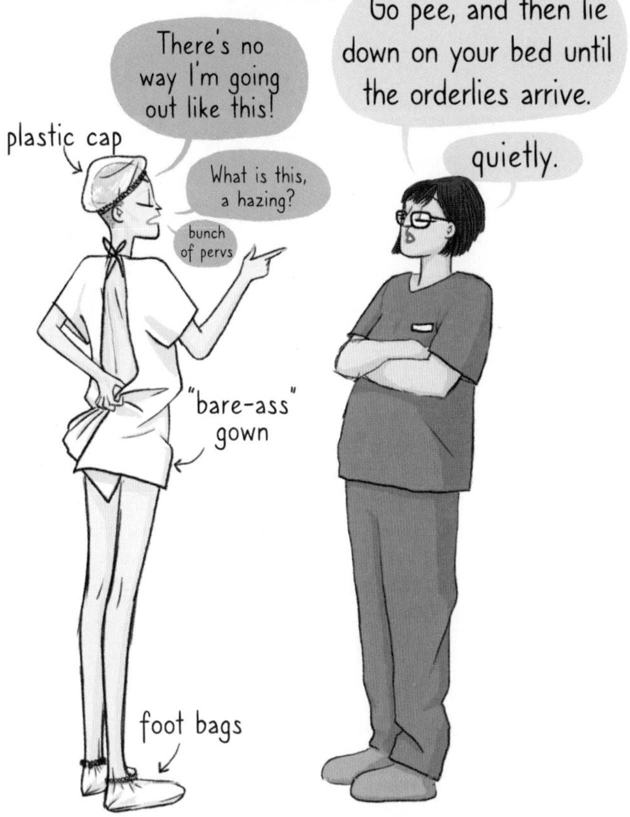

There's no way I'm going out like this!
Go pee, and then lie down on your bed until the orderlies arrive.
quietly.
What is this, a hazing?
bunch of pervs
plastic cap
"bare-ass" gown
foot bags

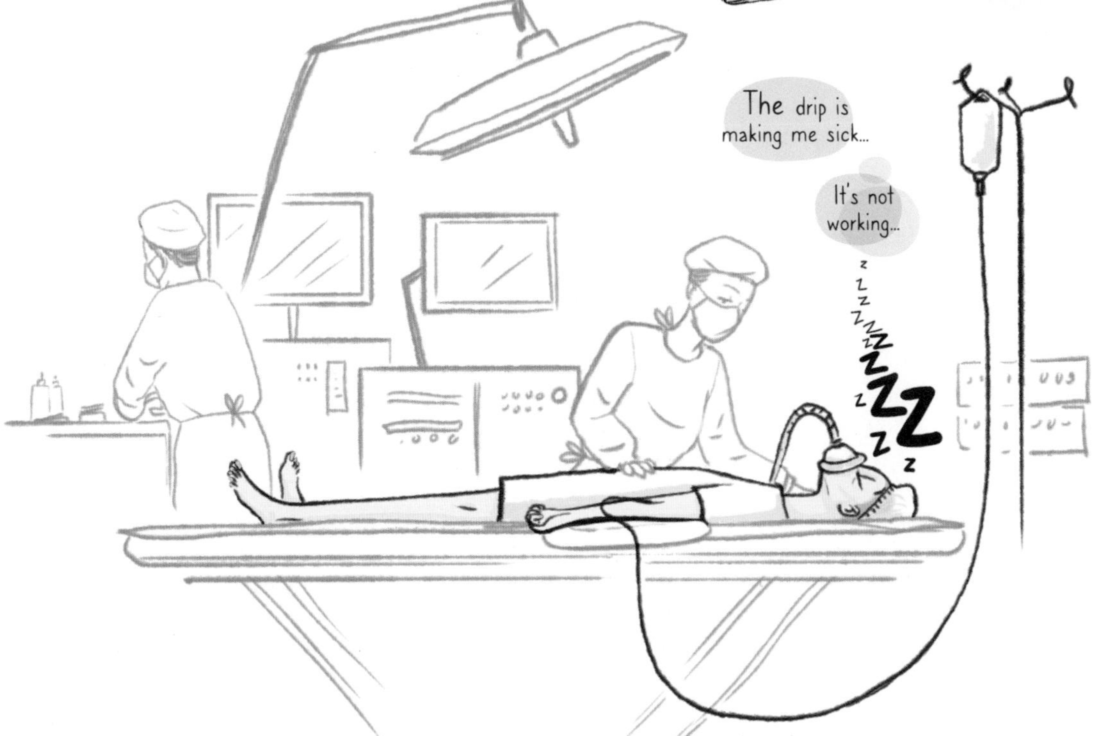

The drip is making me sick...
It's not working...
z z z Z Z Z Z Z z

The operation starts with a coelioscopy. I would've liked to watch, it looks funny: the stomach is inflated with CO_2 to make it like a "bubble" so you can see what you're doing (cut the right part, not leave anything inside, etc.).

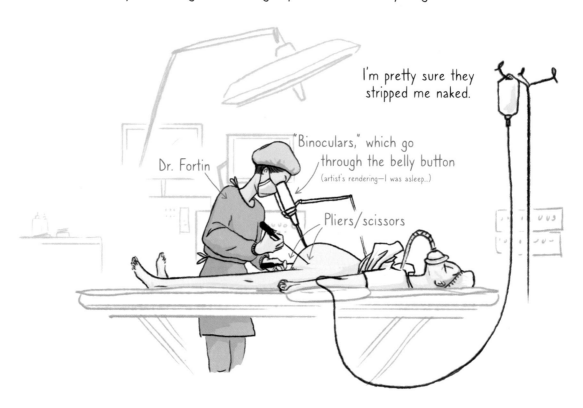

I'm pretty sure they stripped me naked.

Dr. Fortin

"Binoculars," which go through the belly button
(artist's rendering—I was asleep...)

Pliers/scissors

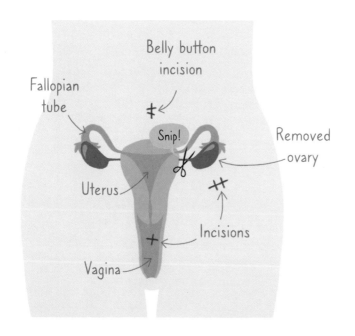

Belly button incision

Fallopian tube

Snip!

Removed ovary

Uterus

Incisions

Vagina

After the operation, the CO_2 inflating the stomach is expelled through the body (thanks to gas exchange with the blood).

Or else a medical student is tasked with pressing on the stomach to deflate it like a balloon. I like this proposition.

In an hour it's all over, and I spend the rest of the day knocked out, occasionally waking up, each time for a little longer.

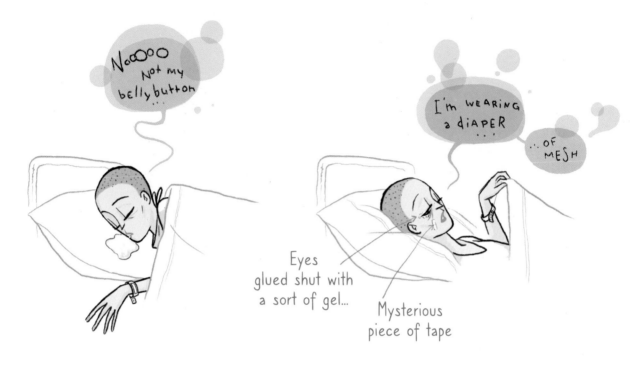

NoOOoo Not my belly button ...

I'm WEARING a diAPER ...
... OF MESH
Eyes glued shut with a sort of gel...
Mysterious piece of tape

THE NEXT DAY, I'M OUT!

I have to wear support stockings and do daily injections of an anticoagulant for a week, so as to avoid any risk of venous thrombosis or pulmonary embolism.

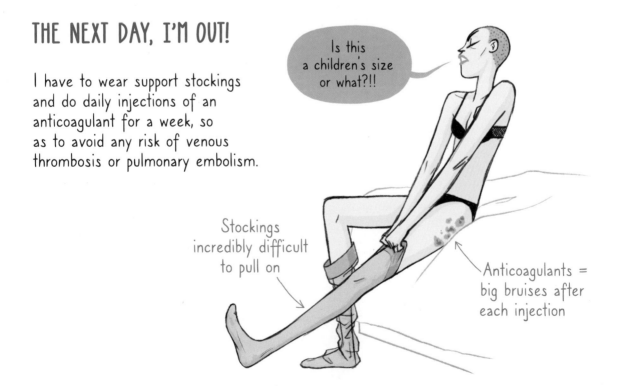

Is this a children's size or what?!!
Stockings incredibly difficult to pull on
Anticoagulants = big bruises after each injection

THE FEEL-GOOD METHOD

MARCH 9 SECOND CONSOLIDATION CHEMO

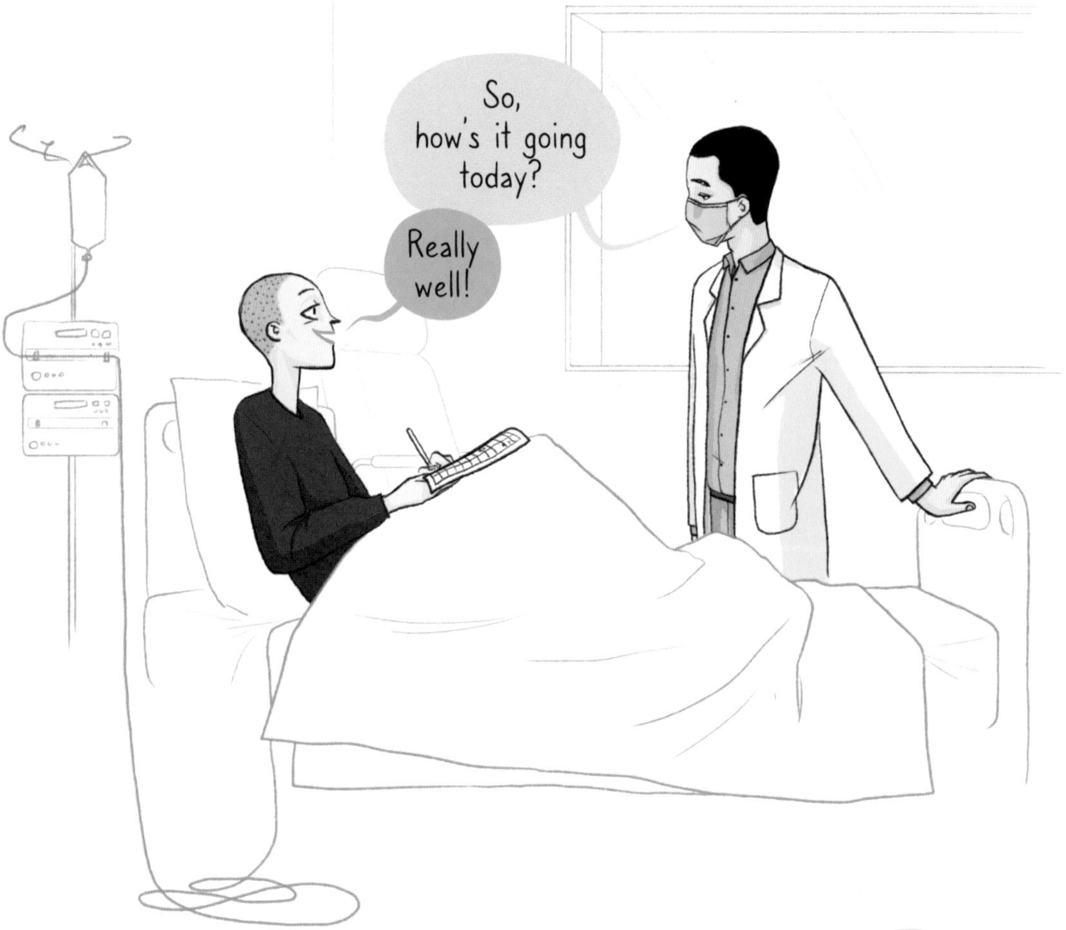
So, how's it going today?
Really well!

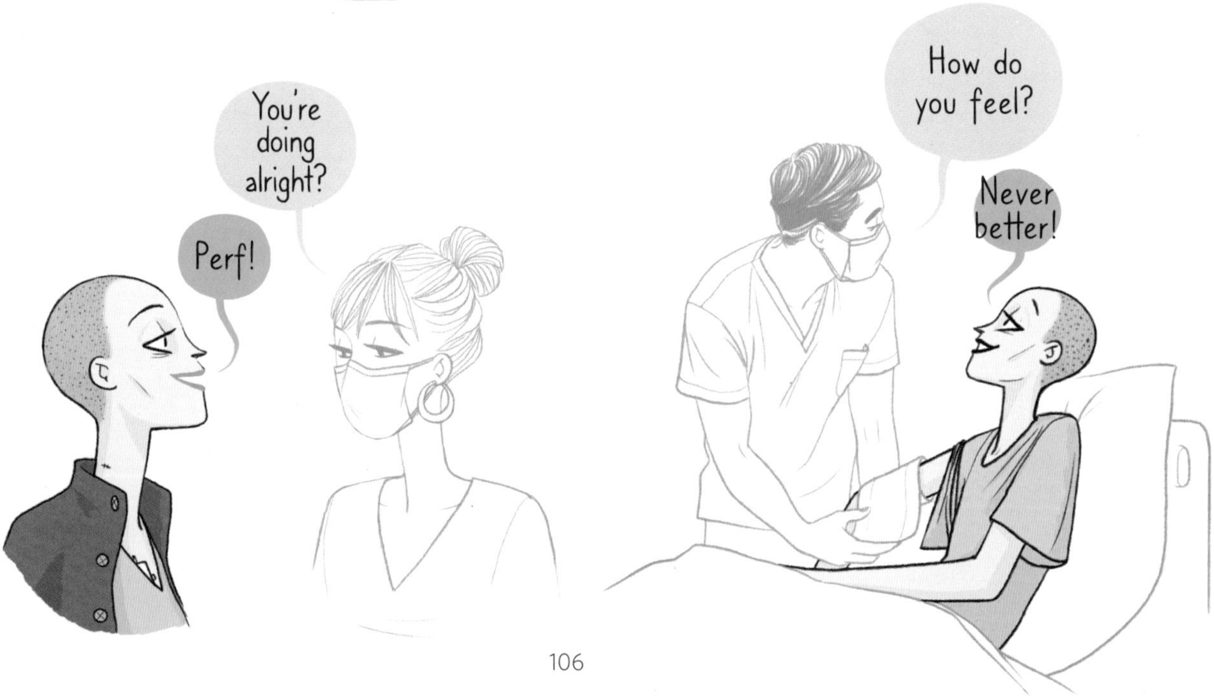
You're doing alright?
Perf!
How do you feel?
Never better!

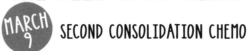

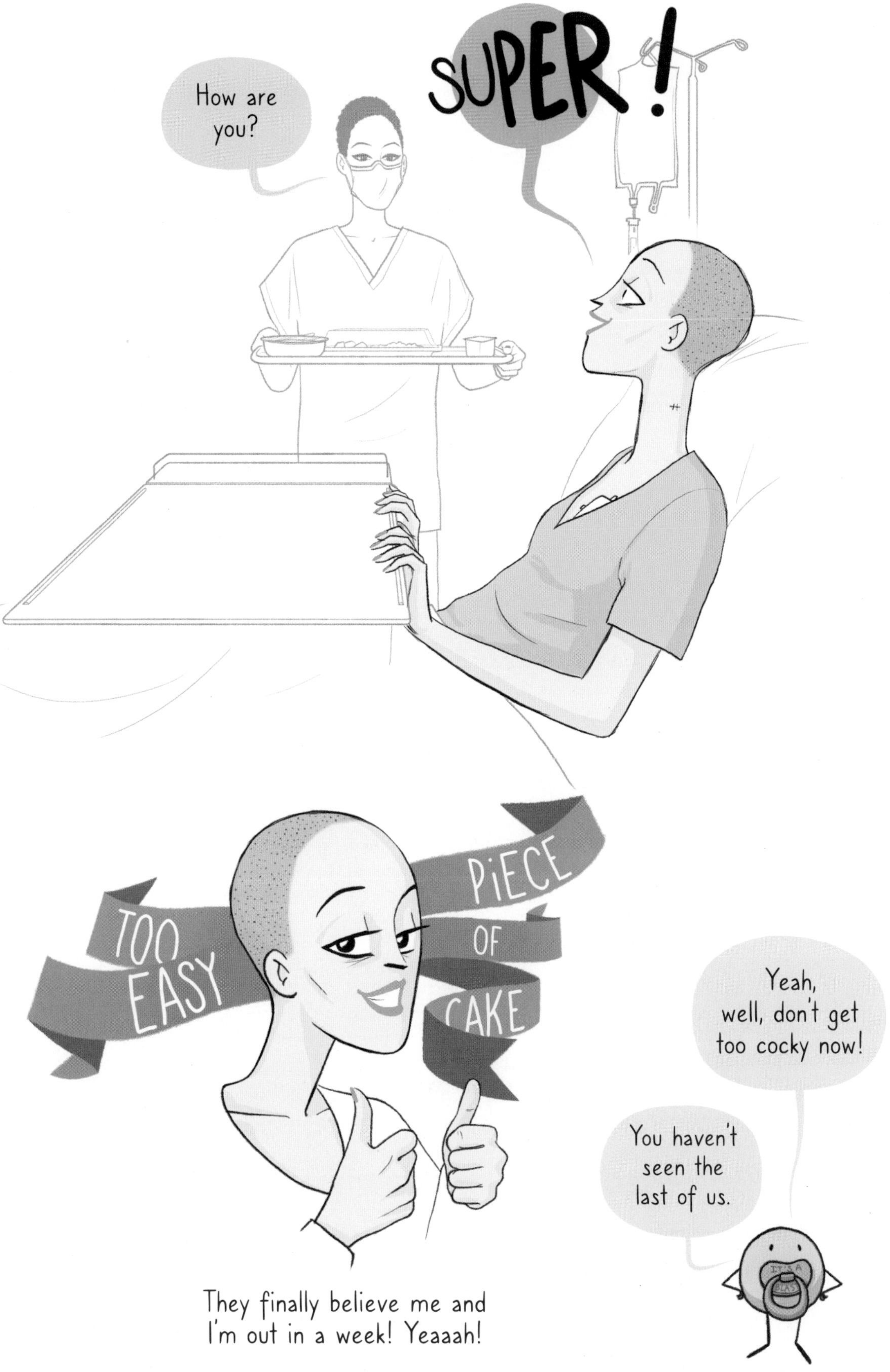
How are you?
SUPER!
TOO EASY
PiECE OF CAKE
They finally believe me and I'm out in a week! Yeaaah!
Yeah, well, don't get too cocky now!
You haven't seen the last of us.

HAZARDS

Appointment next month for the third round of consolidation.
But then two weeks later...

Ms. Pioli? This is the hospital. Your blood tests from yesterday don't look good. You'll need to come back to the hospital.
Are you sure?

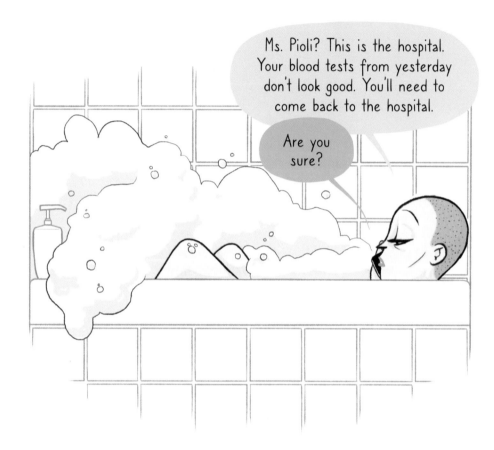

They were sure... It turns out that my numbers were **TERRIBLE!**

	HEMOGLOBIN	WHITE BLOOD CELLS	PLATELETS
BASE VALUES →	between 12 and 16 g/dL	between 4,000 and 11,000/mm^3	between 150,000 and 400,000/mm^3

MY SCORE

Feeling lonely, eh?
What about you, losers?
Haaaaa! What a shit score!
8.4 g/dL
1,600 per mm3
67,000 per mm3
HAHAHA
We're still heeeeere!!!

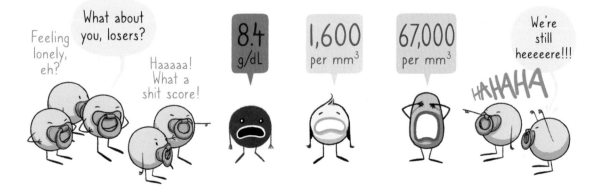

Return to the hospital... I'm pumped full of Zarzio, a growth factor that boosts the production of marrow (red and white blood cells and platelets). I thought it would just take a couple of days, but no! My white blood cells are starting to increase in number, but not all of them: it's specifically the lymphocytes that are proliferating, not the polynuclears. It turns out that there are several types of white blood cells, and each one plays a particular role.

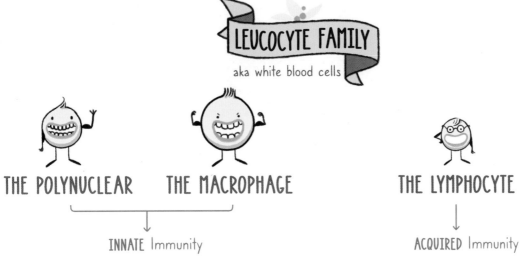

LEUCOCYTE FAMILY

aka white blood cells

THE POLYNUCLEAR   **THE MACROPHAGE**   **THE LYMPHOCYTE**

INNATE Immunity   ACQUIRED Immunity

They gobble up anything **SUSPICIOUS** (foreign or cancerous bodies) in a nonspecific way. The macrophage is larger than the polynuclear, and it also destroys blood cells at the end of their life span, by order of the spleen (now I finally know what it's for!). These two act quickly during an infection, sort of like a surveillance patrol.

This one's smaller than the other two but can "**LEARN**": when we get vaccinated, we teach it to recognize any future threats (flu, tetanus, etc.) and to produce antibodies to fight the threat. It acts in a specific manner: if it spots anything suspicious that it doesn't understand, it just goes on its way. So when we get sick, the polynuclears and macrophages run the show, and the lymphocyte learns its lesson.

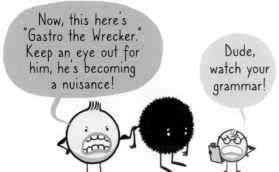

Now, this here's "Gastro the Wrecker." Keep an eye out for him, he's becoming a nuisance!

Dude, watch your grammar!

I went to college, you uncultured swine!

MAYHEM

Despite the Zarzio, the polynuclears continue their free fall.

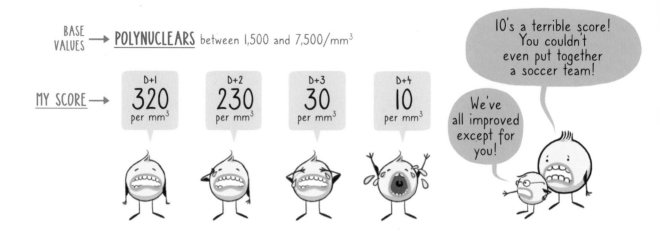

BASE VALUES → **POLYNUCLEARS** between 1,500 and 7,500/mm³

MY SCORE →

D+1
320 per mm³

D+2
230 per mm³

D+3
30 per mm³

D+4
10 per mm³

10's a terrible score! You couldn't even put together a soccer team!

We've all improved except for you!

I'm starting to worry a little, especially since there's nothing that can be done: this isn't like when you're low on iron or vitamins, and you can just swallow some pills and zip! Here we go! With this, you just have to wait, but it's agonizing. And what if it NEVER IMPROVES? Everything's gone way too well until now, to the point that I still don't feel sick. I've always had the impression that I really shouldn't be concerned, that everything will turn out all right because death is something out of the ordinary, exceptional, and could never happen to me. I'm ordinary. There's nothing all that exceptional about me.

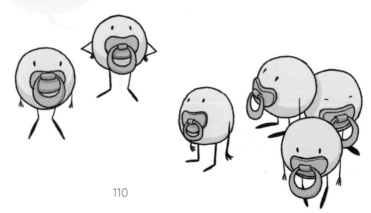

Well, then... I don't know what more we can say...

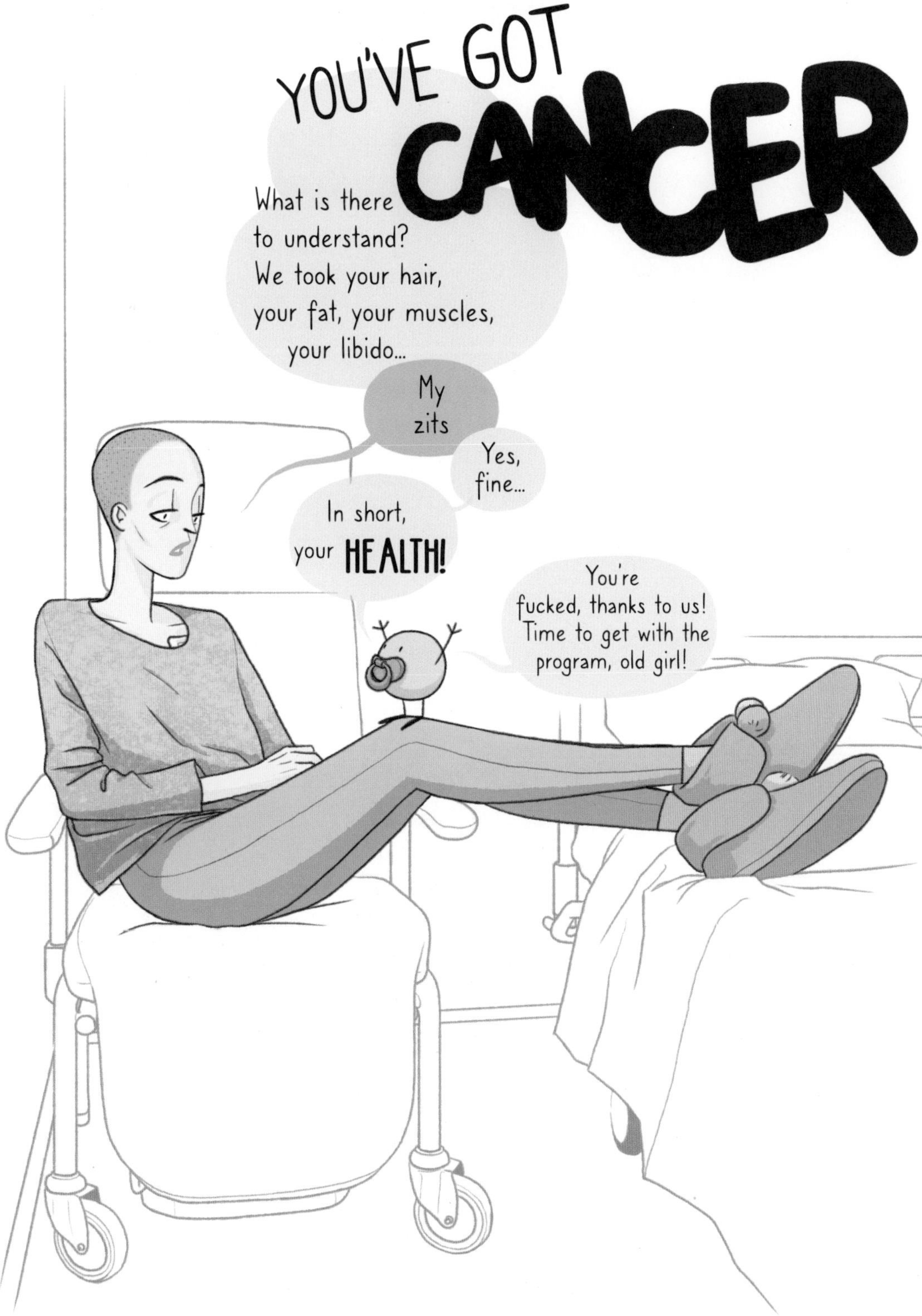
YOU'VE GOT CANCER
What is there to understand? We took your hair, your fat, your muscles, your libido...
My zits
Yes, fine...
In short, your HEALTH!
You're fucked, thanks to us! Time to get with the program, old girl!

It ends up taking 10 days for these damn polynuclears to decide to improve. And all this time is eating into my "vacation time," so I only have about a dozen days of freedom before my third consolidation, which'll be impossible to postpone.

A CHANGE OF SCENERY

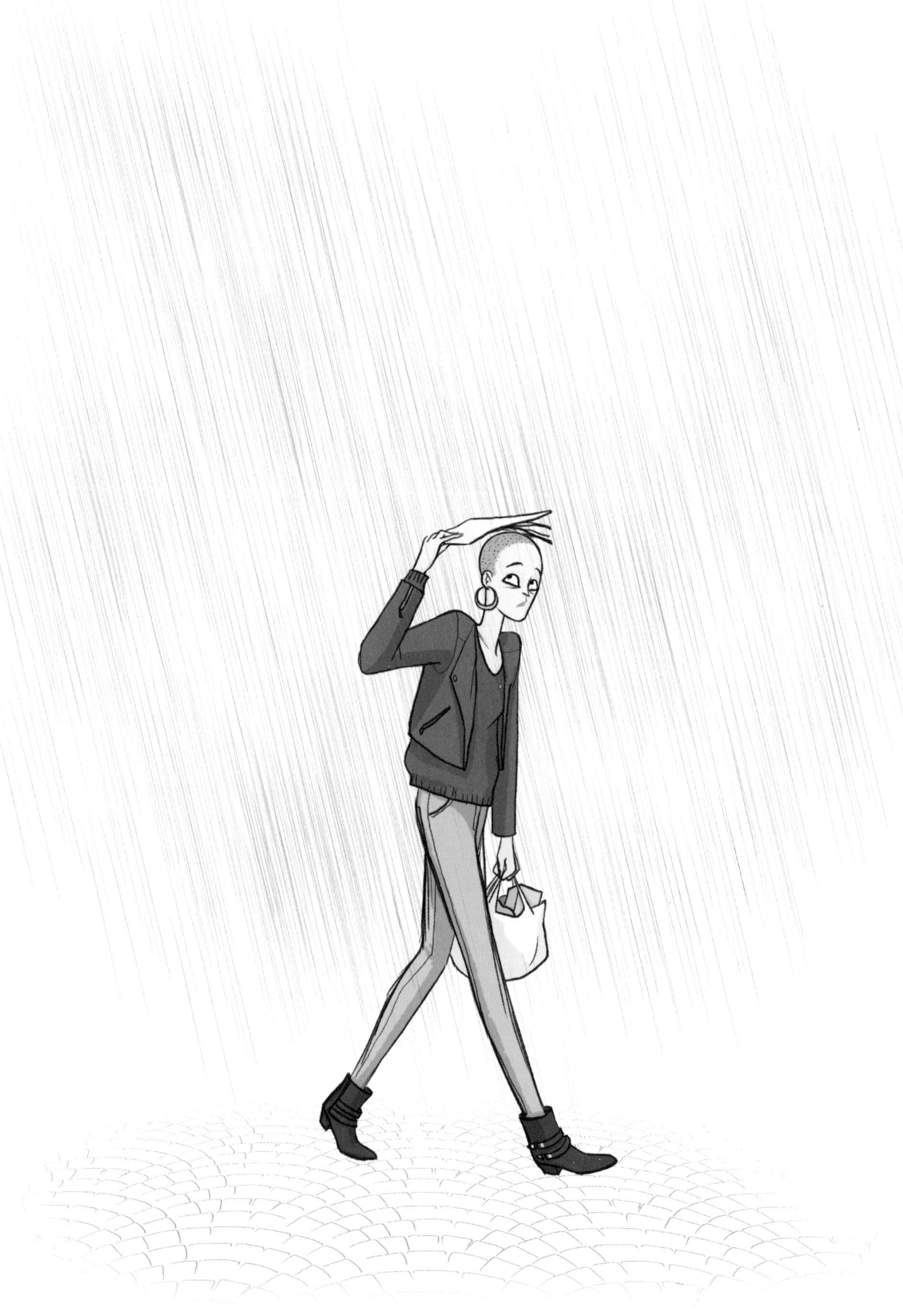

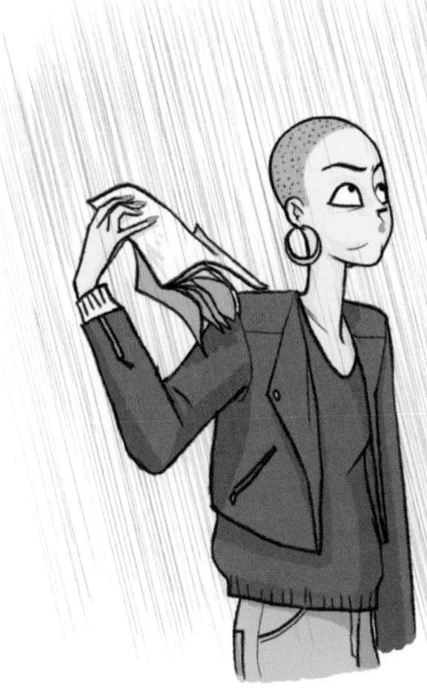

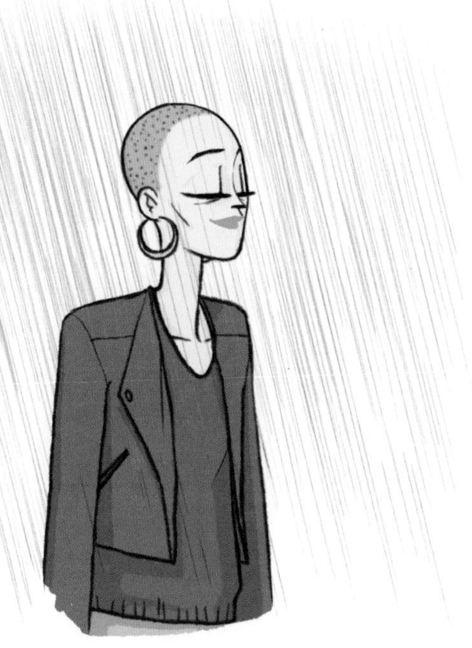

I sometimes think Paris isn't the best
place for rest and relaxation. It's gray,
polluted, full of people, noises, cars.

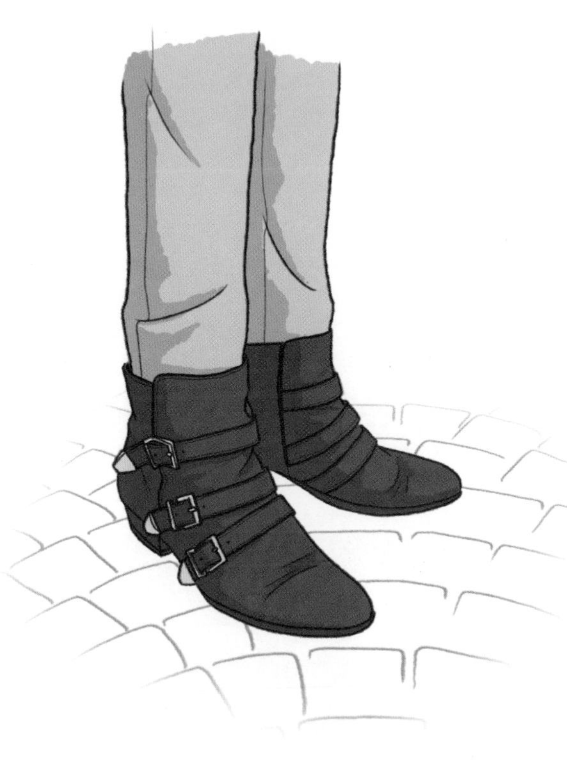

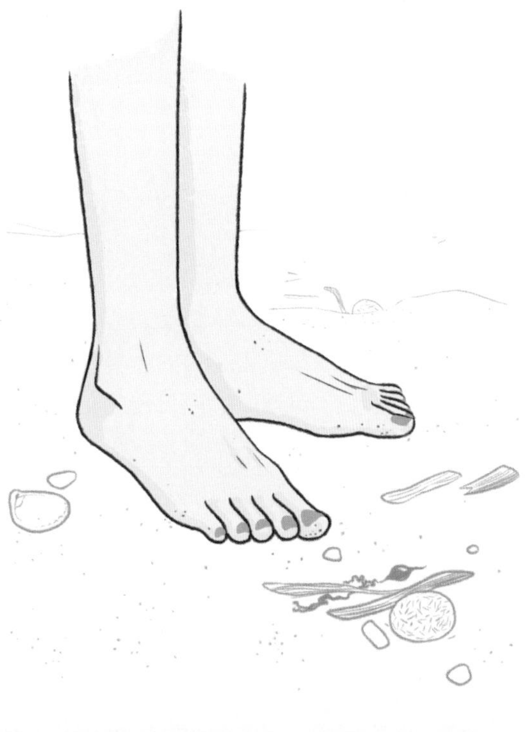

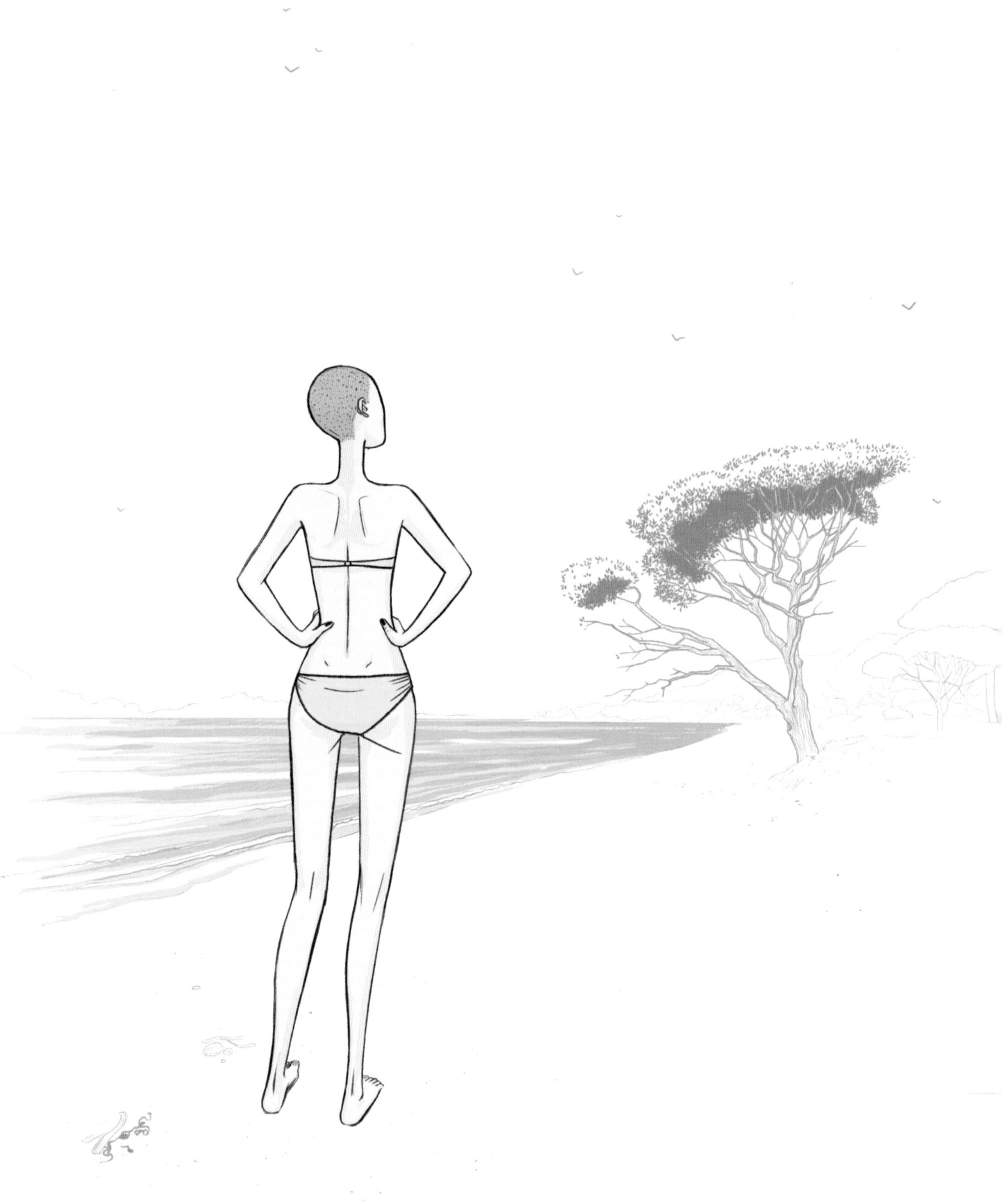

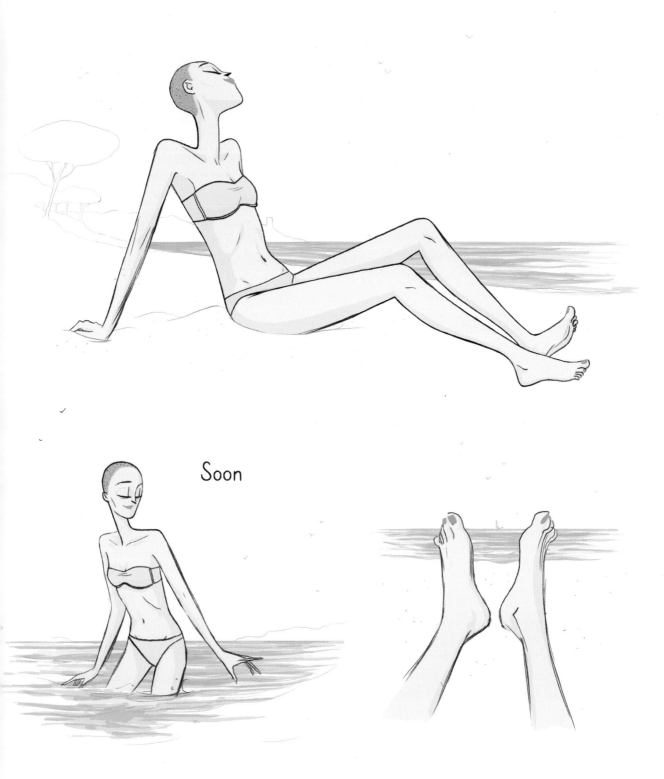

Soon

I'm not allowed to travel for the time being.
I have to stay close to the hospital, in case of an emergency.

SPRING/SUMMER

Paris

Quack

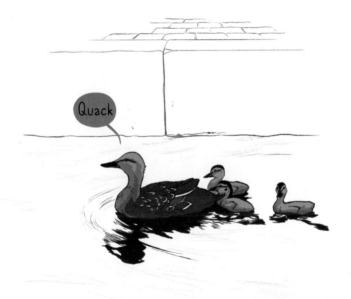

THE GREAT LEAP

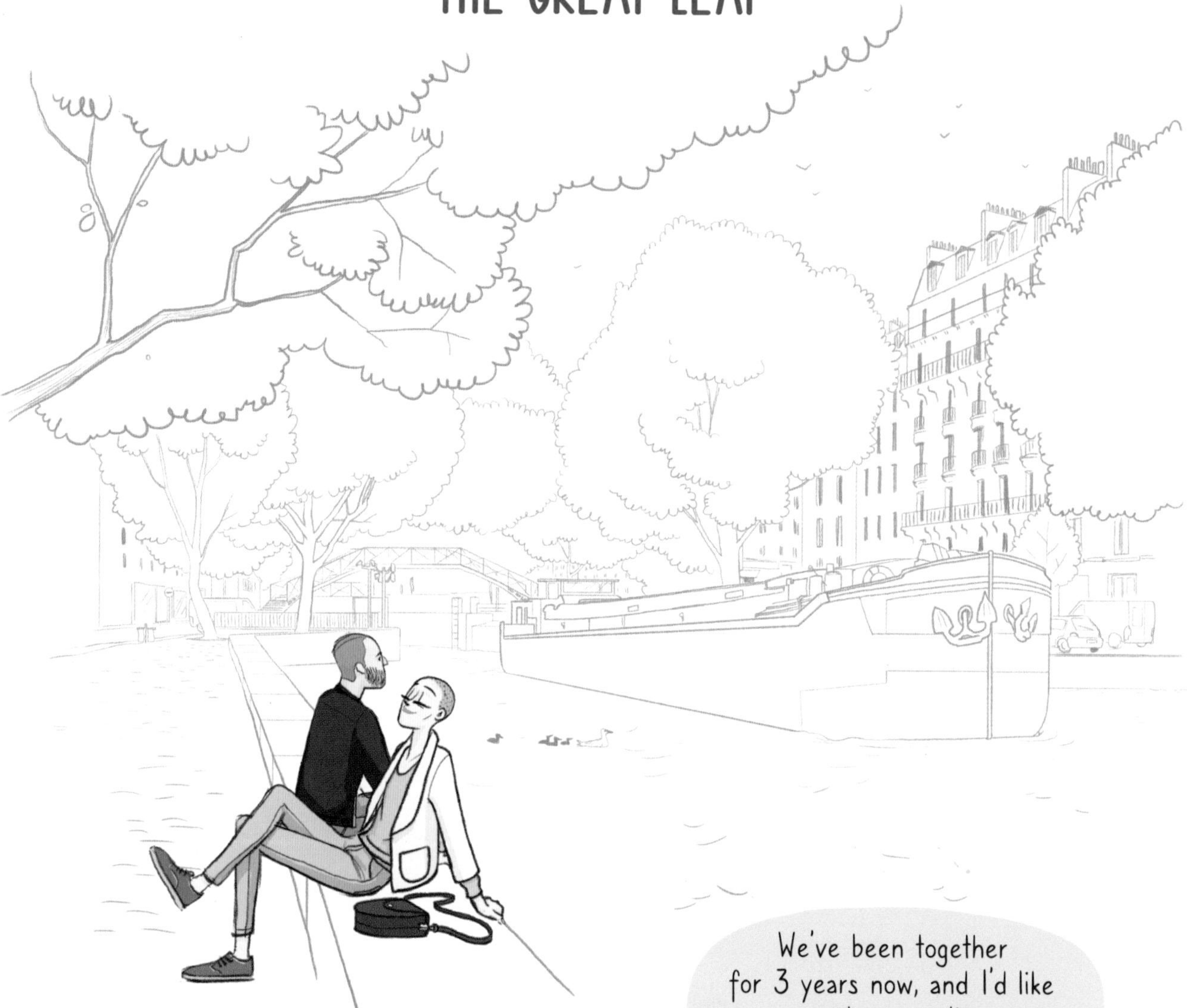

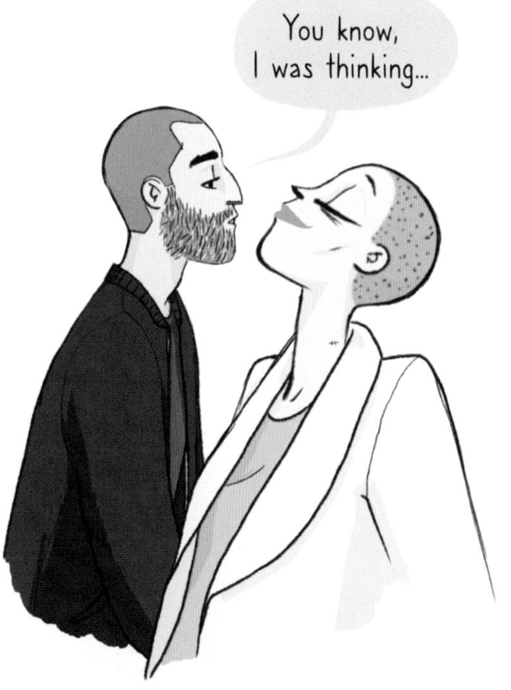
You know, I was thinking...

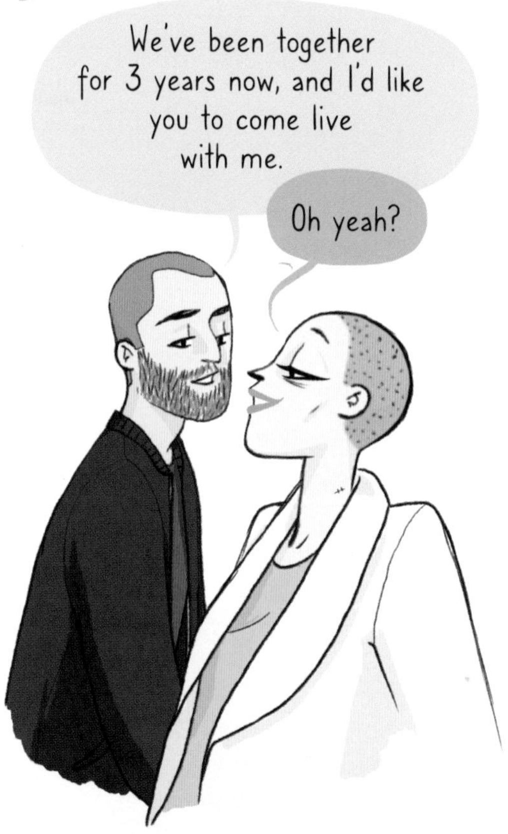
We've been together for 3 years now, and I'd like you to come live with me.
Oh yeah?

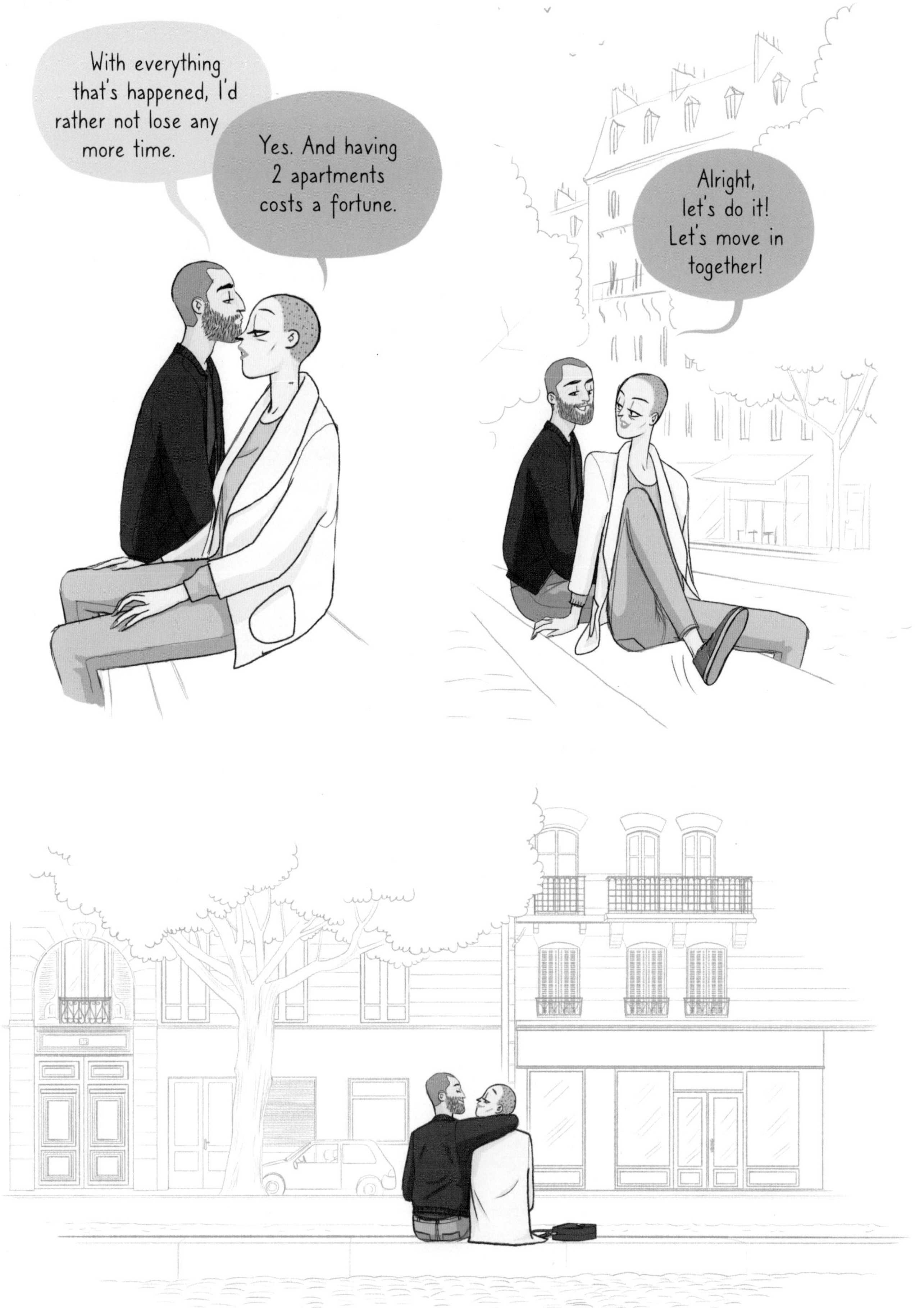
With everything that's happened, I'd rather not lose any more time.
Yes. And having 2 apartments costs a fortune.
Alright, let's do it! Let's move in together!

BATHROOM RHAPSODY

April 9-16: 3rd consolidation. Nothing to report, everything's going well.

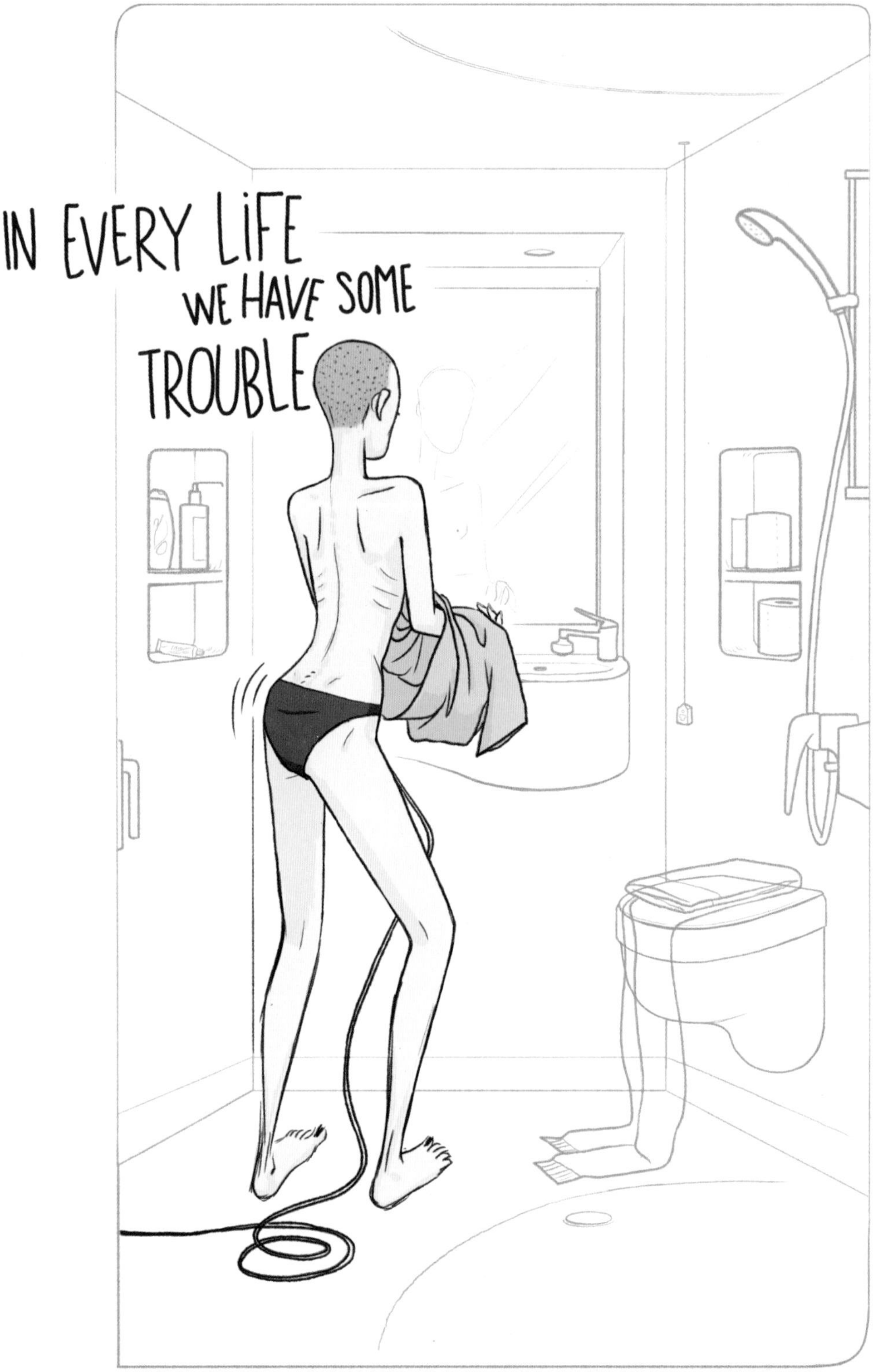
IN EVERY LIFE
WE HAVE SOME
TROUBLE

The bathroom is really just three and a half square feet. It looks like a plastic teleportation booth, where you can take a shower while sitting on the toilet.

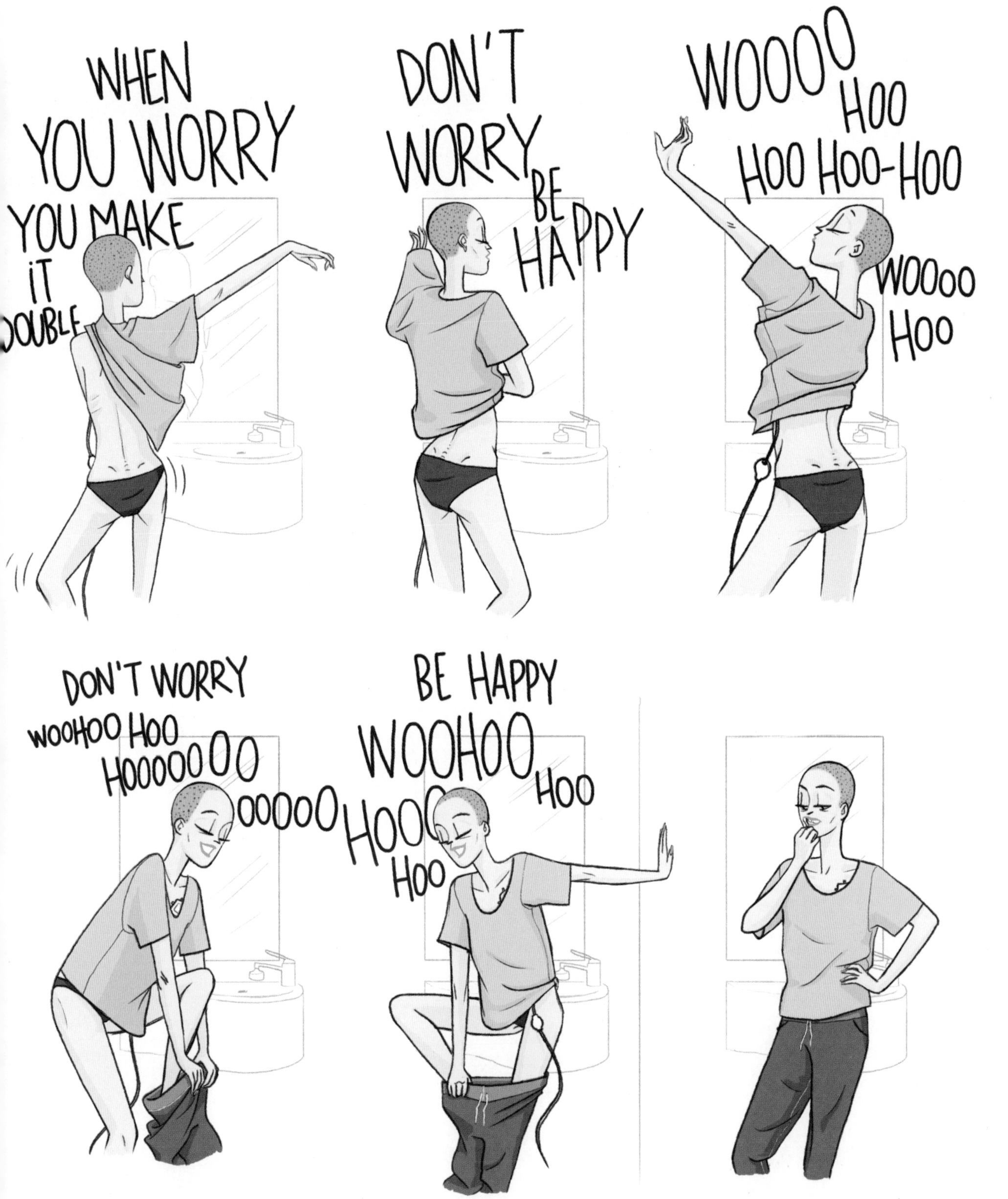
WHEN YOU WORRY YOU MAKE iT DOUBLE
DON'T WORRY BE HAPPY
WOOOO HOO HOO HOO-HOO
WOOOO HOO
DON'T WORRY
WOOHOO HOO HOOOOOOO OOOOO
BE HAPPY
WOOHOO HOO HOOO HOO

Considering the situation, is my subconscious trying to send me a message?

PUBLIC DOMAIN

I've been sick for almost 6 months, and so, inevitably, I get asked the same questions over and over.

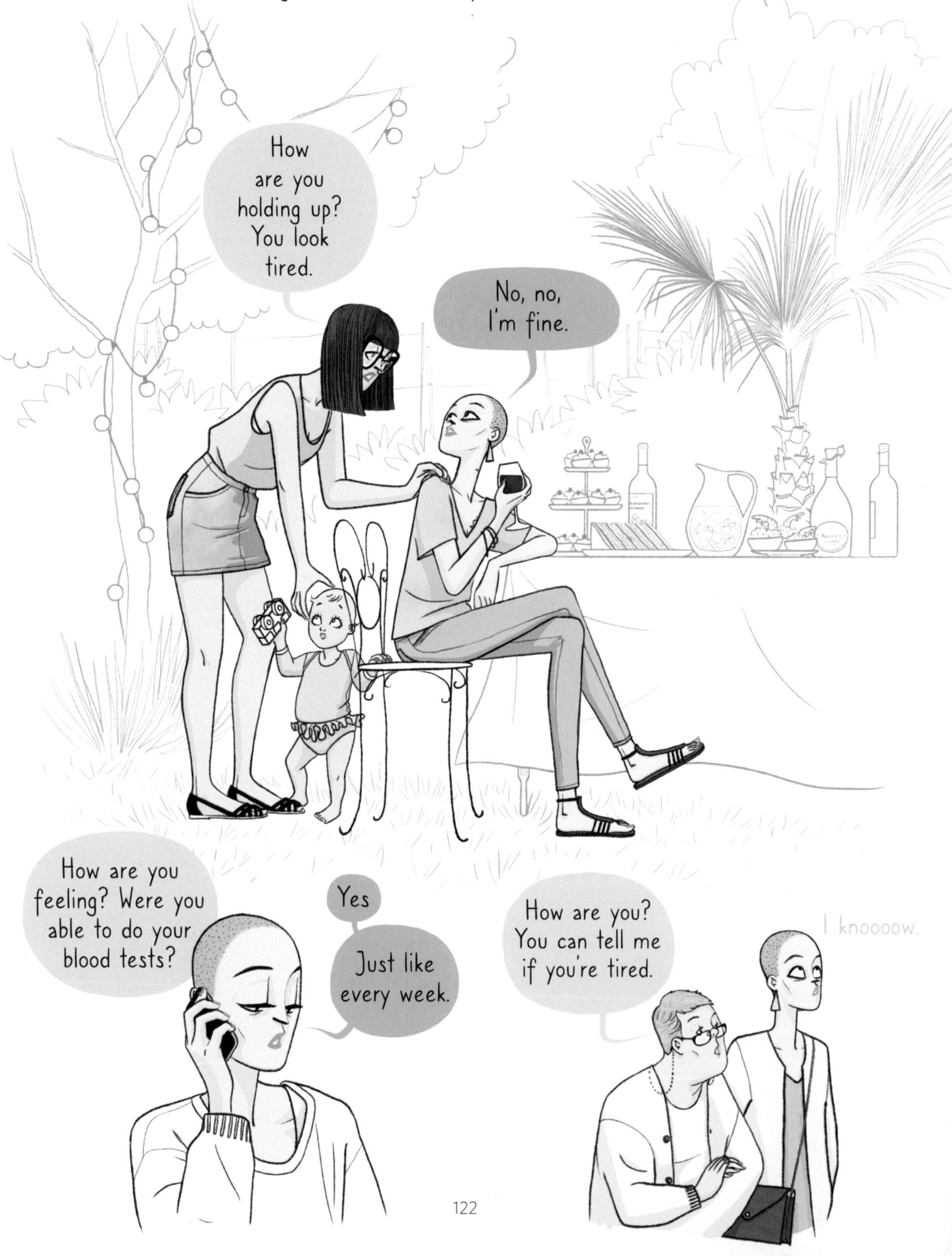
How are you holding up? You look tired.
No, no, I'm fine.
How are you feeling? Were you able to do your blood tests?
Yes
Just like every week.
How are you? You can tell me if you're tired.
I knooooow.

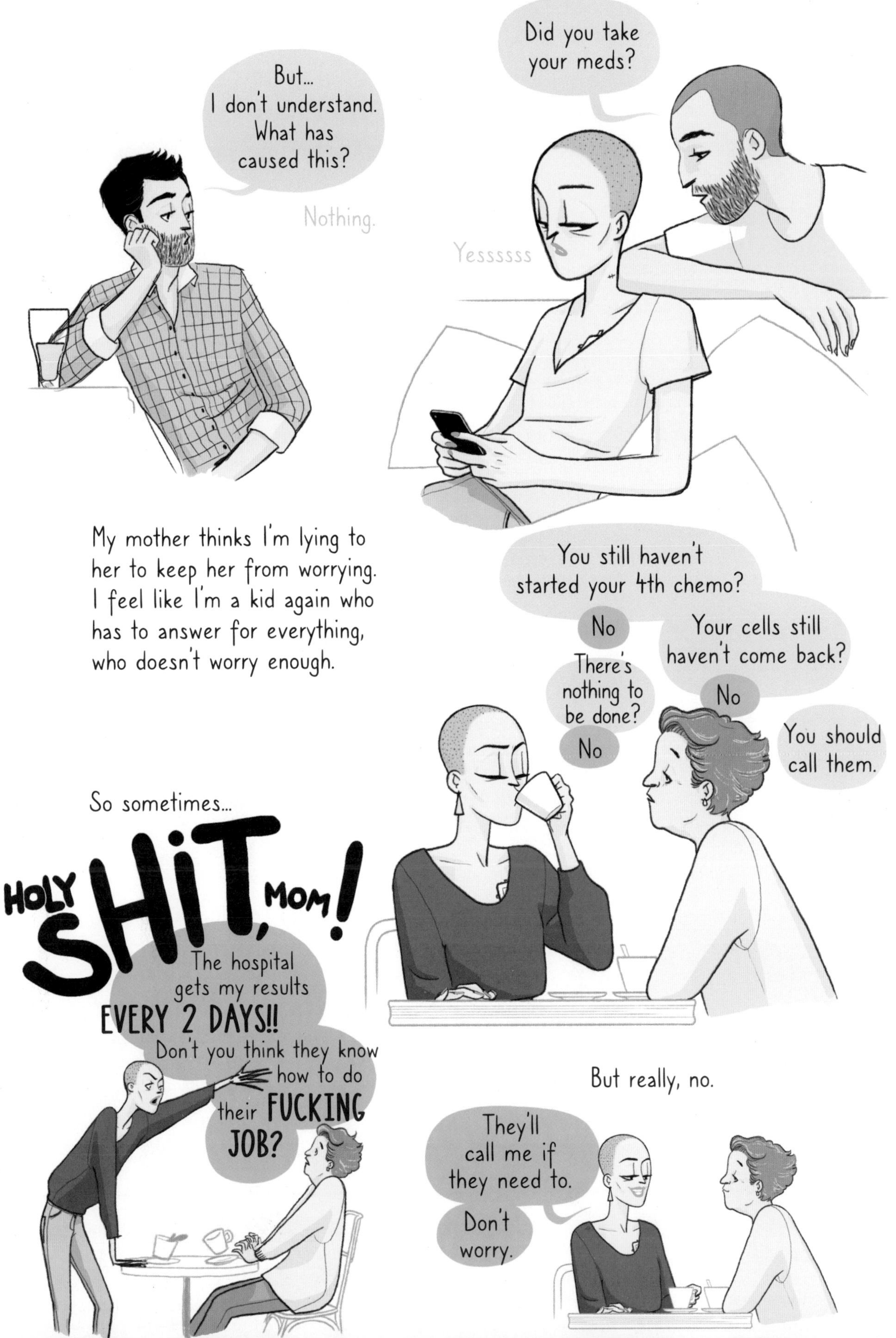
But... I don't understand. What has caused this?
Nothing.
Did you take your meds?
Yessssss
My mother thinks I'm lying to her to keep her from worrying. I feel like I'm a kid again who has to answer for everything, who doesn't worry enough.
You still haven't started your 4th chemo?
No
Your cells still haven't come back?
No
There's nothing to be done?
No
You should call them.
So sometimes...
HOLY SHIT, MOM!
The hospital gets my results EVERY 2 DAYS!!
Don't you think they know how to do their FUCKING JOB?
But really, no.
They'll call me if they need to.
Don't worry.

A CARDBOARD BODY

Time passes and still no 4th consolidation chemo. My blood tests aren't great, and I have aplasia, so we can't start chemo again until I improve. So while waiting, I pack. I'll be moving out at the end of May.

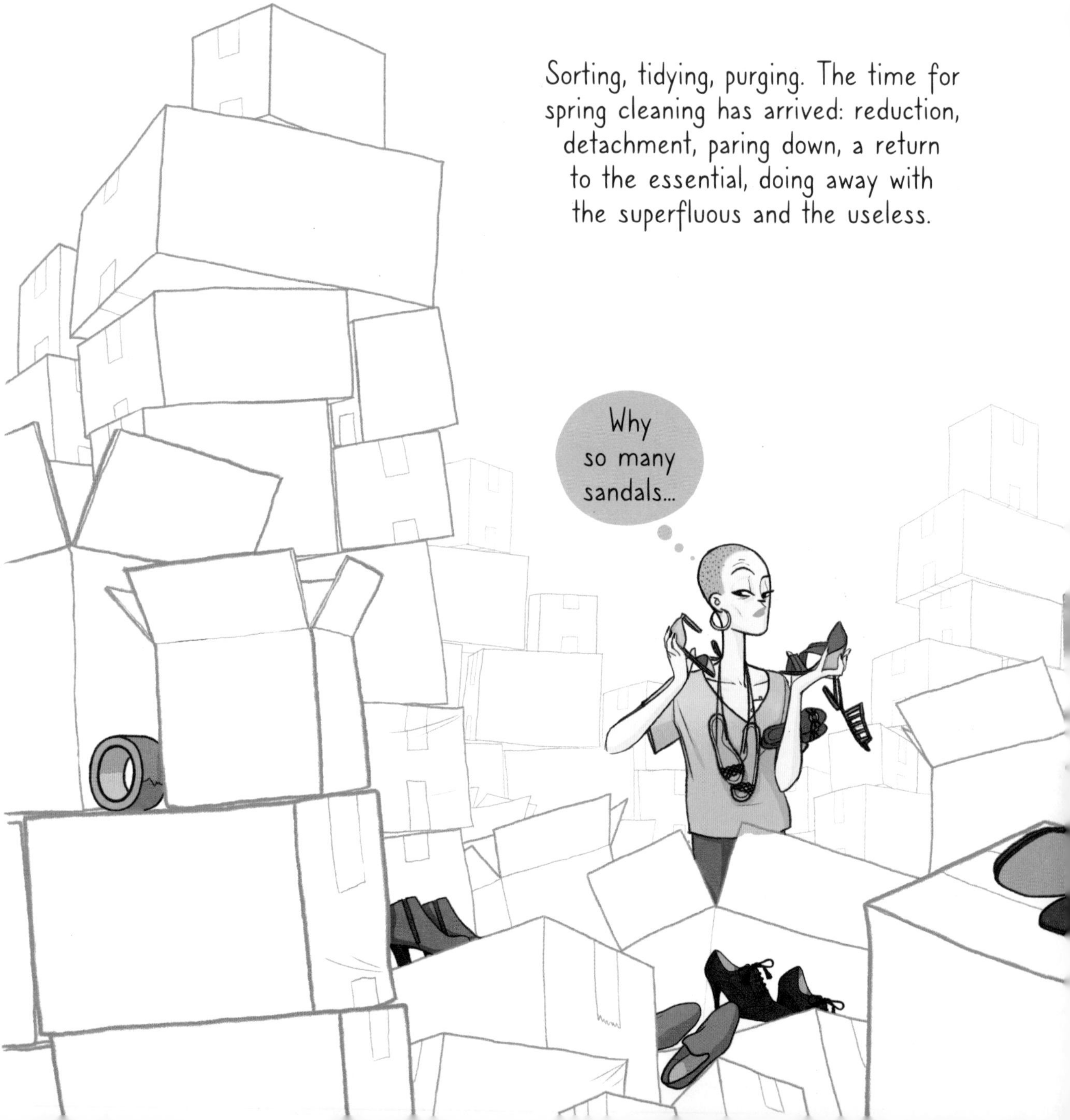
Sorting, tidying, purging. The time for spring cleaning has arrived: reduction, detachment, paring down, a return to the essential, doing away with the superfluous and the useless.
Why so many sandals...

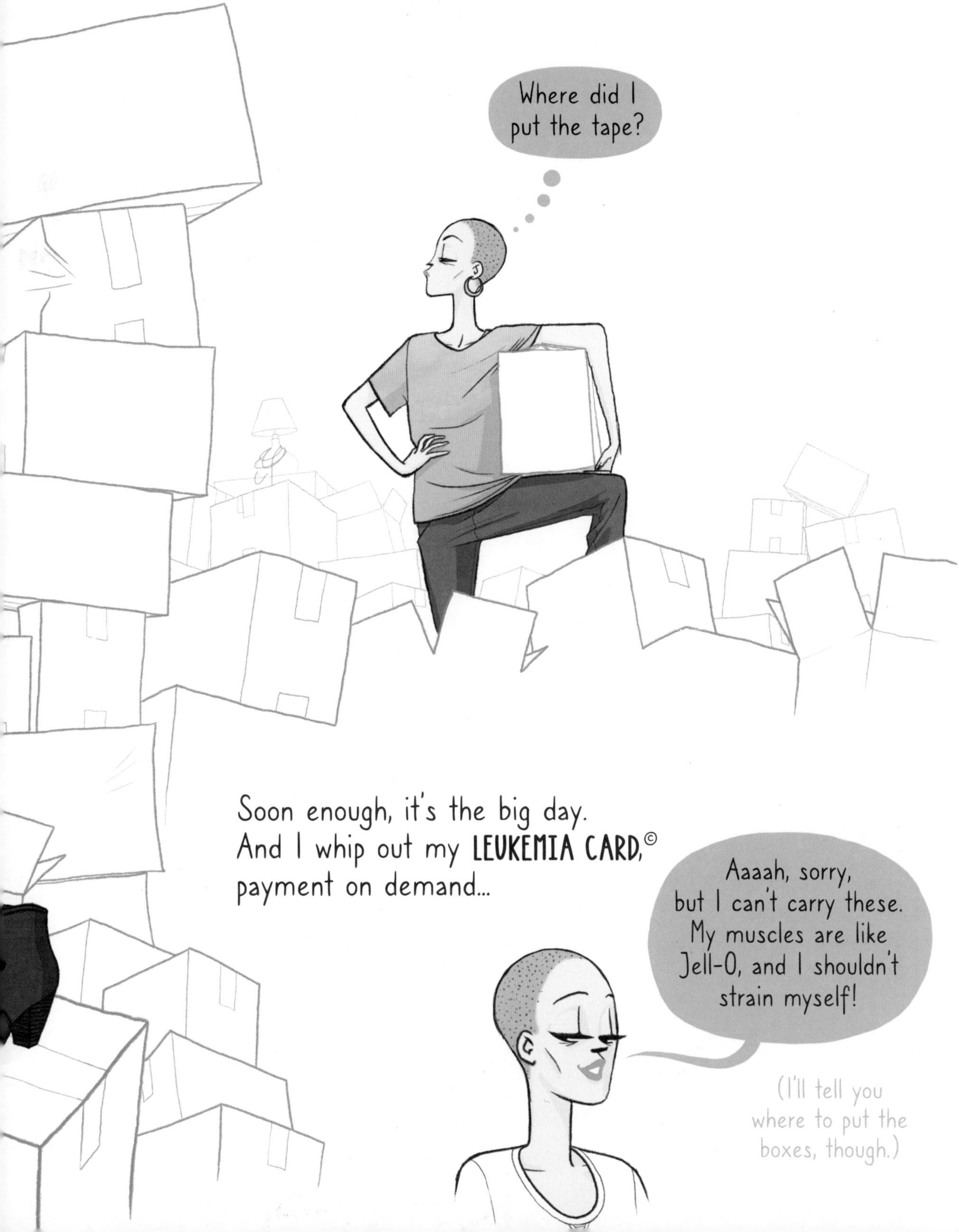
Where did I put the tape?
Soon enough, it's the big day. And I whip out my LEUKEMIA CARD,© payment on demand...
Aaaah, sorry, but I can't carry these. My muscles are like Jell-O, and I shouldn't strain myself!
(I'll tell you where to put the boxes, though.)

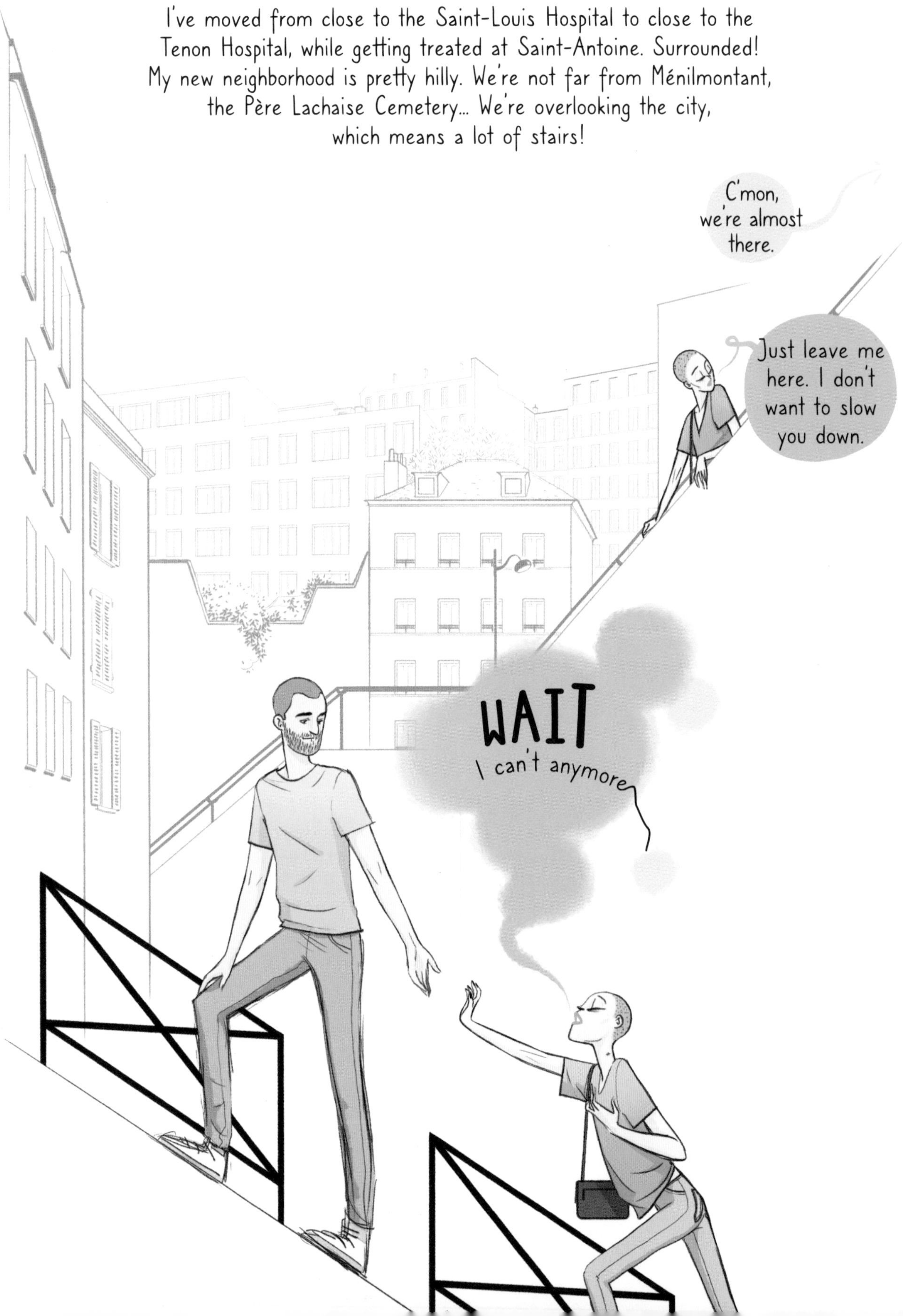
I've moved from close to the Saint-Louis Hospital to close to the Tenon Hospital, while getting treated at Saint-Antoine. Surrounded! My new neighborhood is pretty hilly. We're not far from Ménilmontant, the Père Lachaise Cemetery... We're overlooking the city, which means a lot of stairs!
C'mon, we're almost there.
Just leave me here. I don't want to slow you down.
WAIT
I can't anymore

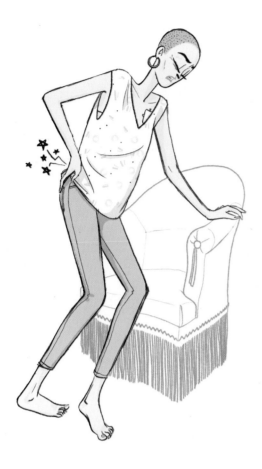

I now live on the 6th floor, without an elevator. I don't know if it's connected, but my muscles feel rusty. Especially in my legs.

Standing up after sitting for a while has become difficult. I feel like my thigh and calf muscles have shrunk.

Look!!! You can CLEARLY SEE that my muscles are SHORTER!
I'll remind you that you've never been able to touch your toes.

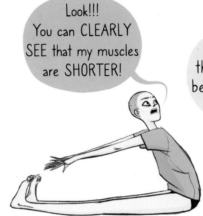

And my eyes are becoming dry and sensitive...

Really, there's a grain of sand in there, I can feel it!
No... I don't see anything.

... and I come down with a raging case of sinusitis from a simple cold.

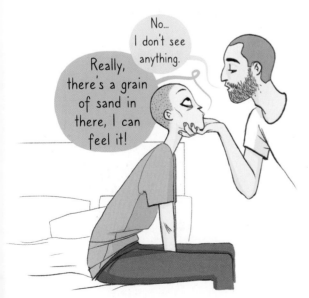

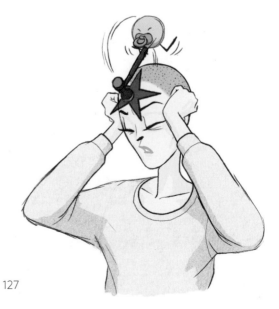

FOLLICULARLY CHALLENGED

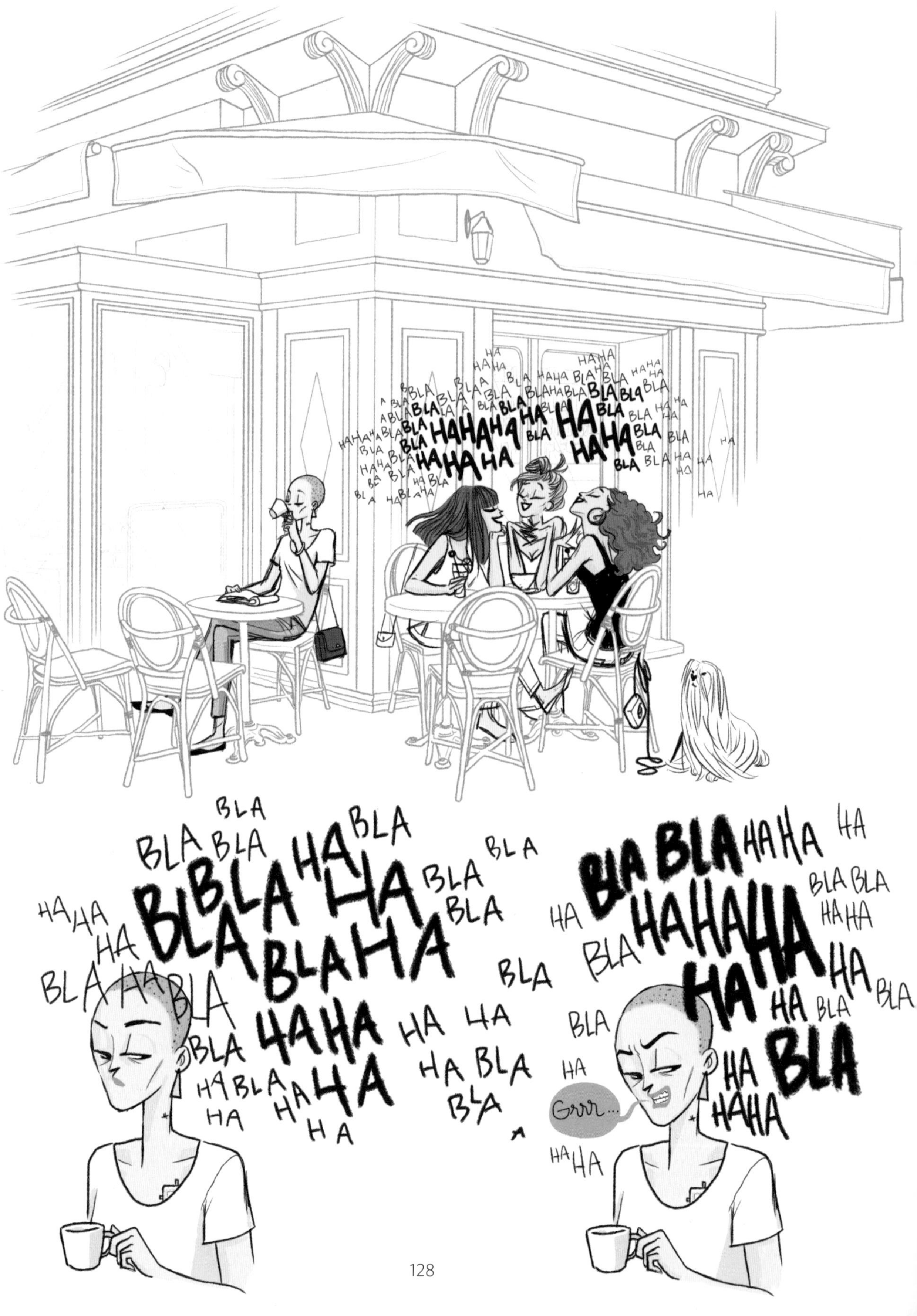
Grrr...

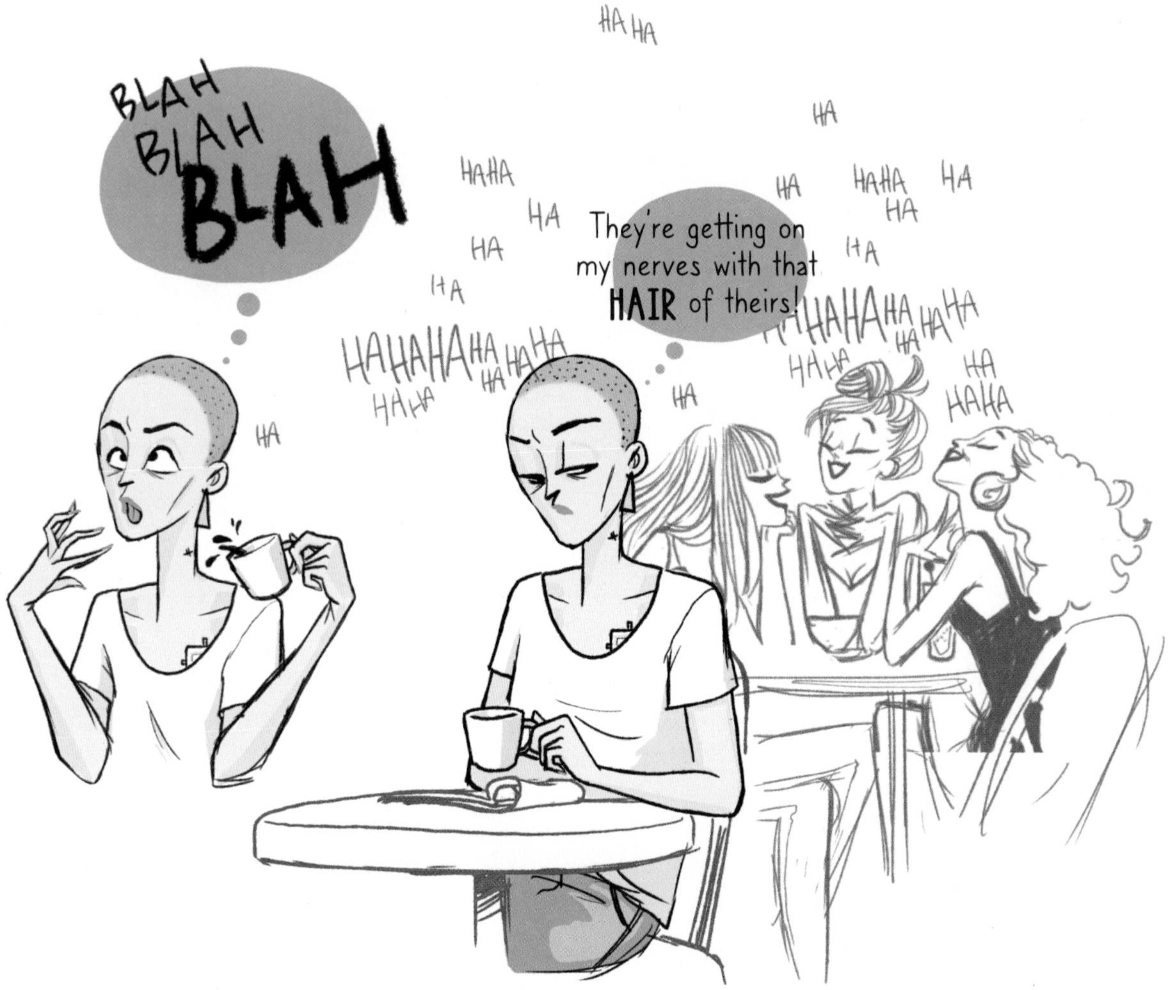
BLAH BLAH BLAH
They're getting on my nerves with that HAIR of theirs!
HAHAHAHA HA HA
HAHA
HAHAHAHA HA HA HA

When my hair starts to grow back, I look like a dandelion.

So I shave it regularly.

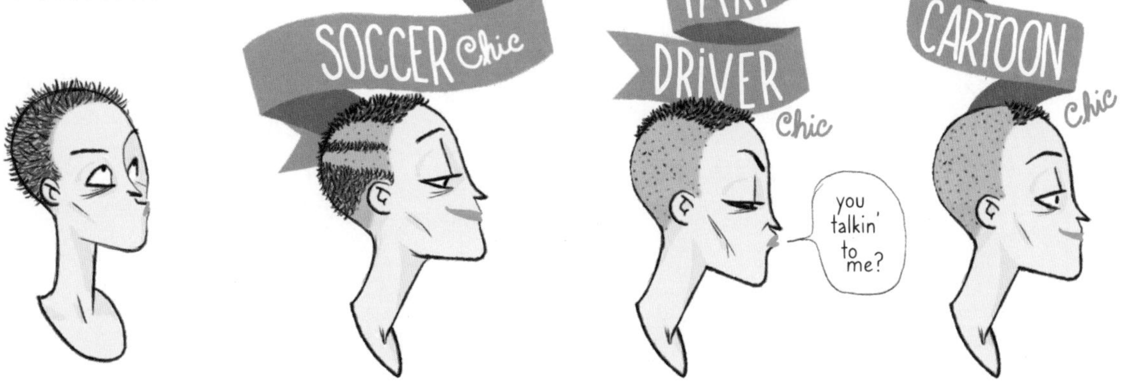
SOCCER Chic
TAXI DRIVER Chic
you talkin' to me?
CARTOON Chic

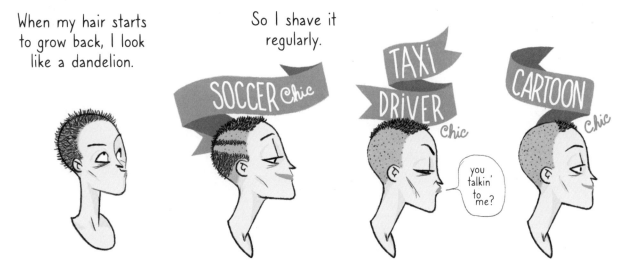

It's going to be a long while before I can get a real haircut again.
It's really not fair. I have to steel myself to be patient.

OTHER THAN THAT I'M FINE

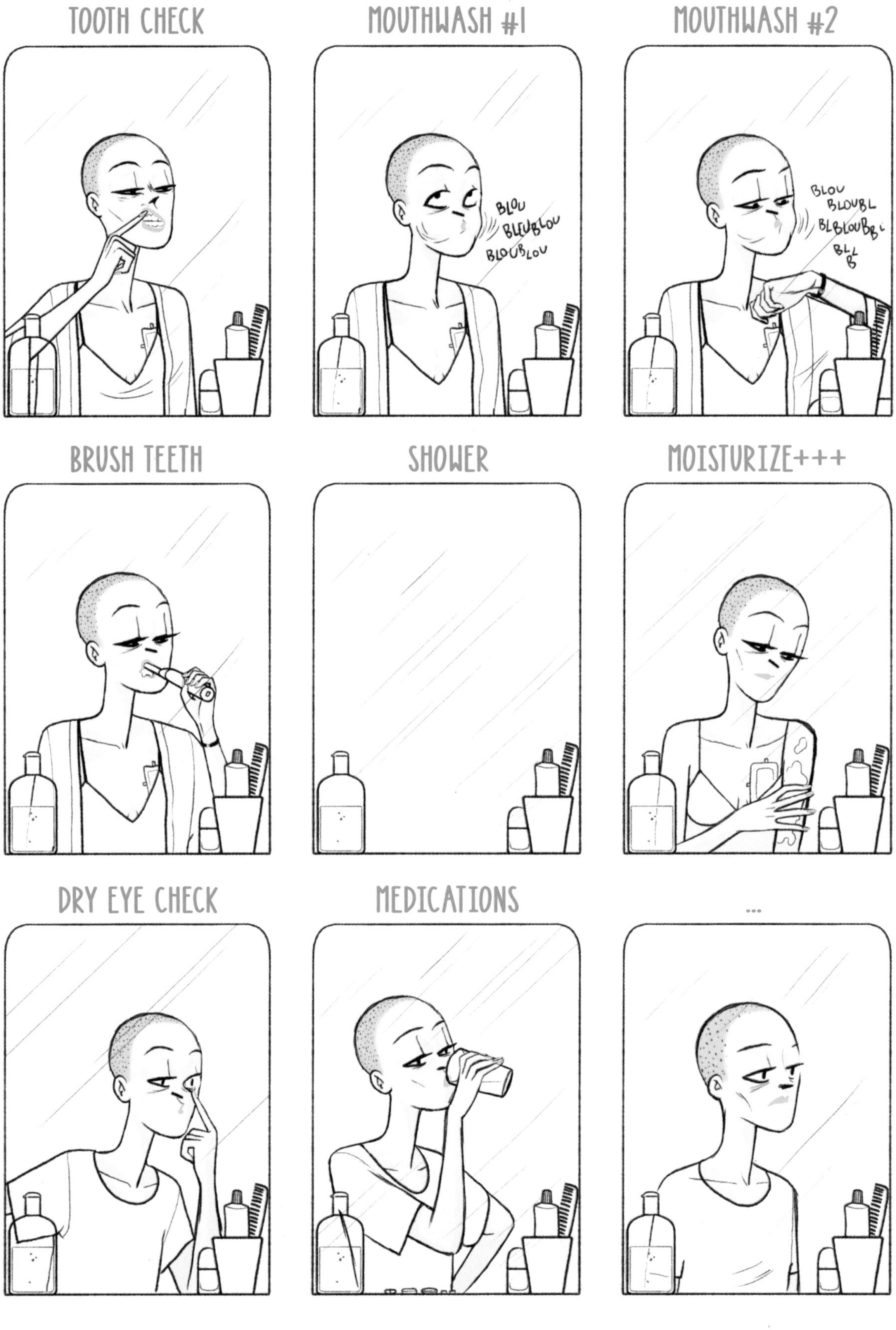
TOOTH CHECK
MOUTHWASH #1
BLOU
BLEUBLOU
BLOUBLOU
MOUTHWASH #2
BLOU
BLOUBL
BRUSH TEETH
SHOWER
MOISTURIZE+++
DRY EYE CHECK
MEDICATIONS
...

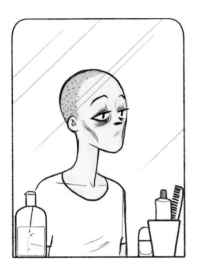
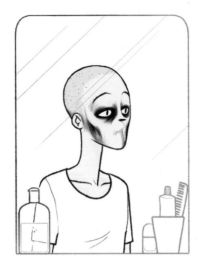
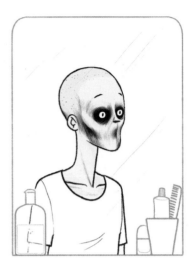
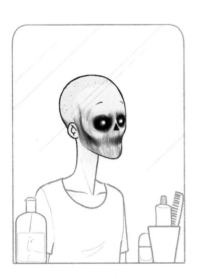

I feel like
my body is
degrading,
crumbling,
deteriorating,
little by little.

This is no longer
me. Just a list
of things to do
to slow the damage,
a betrayal.

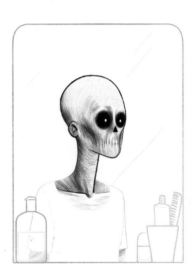
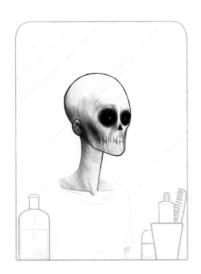
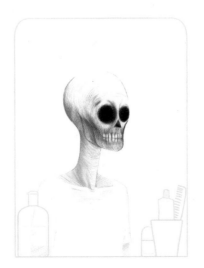
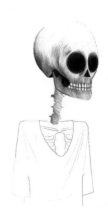

ILLUSIONS

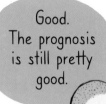

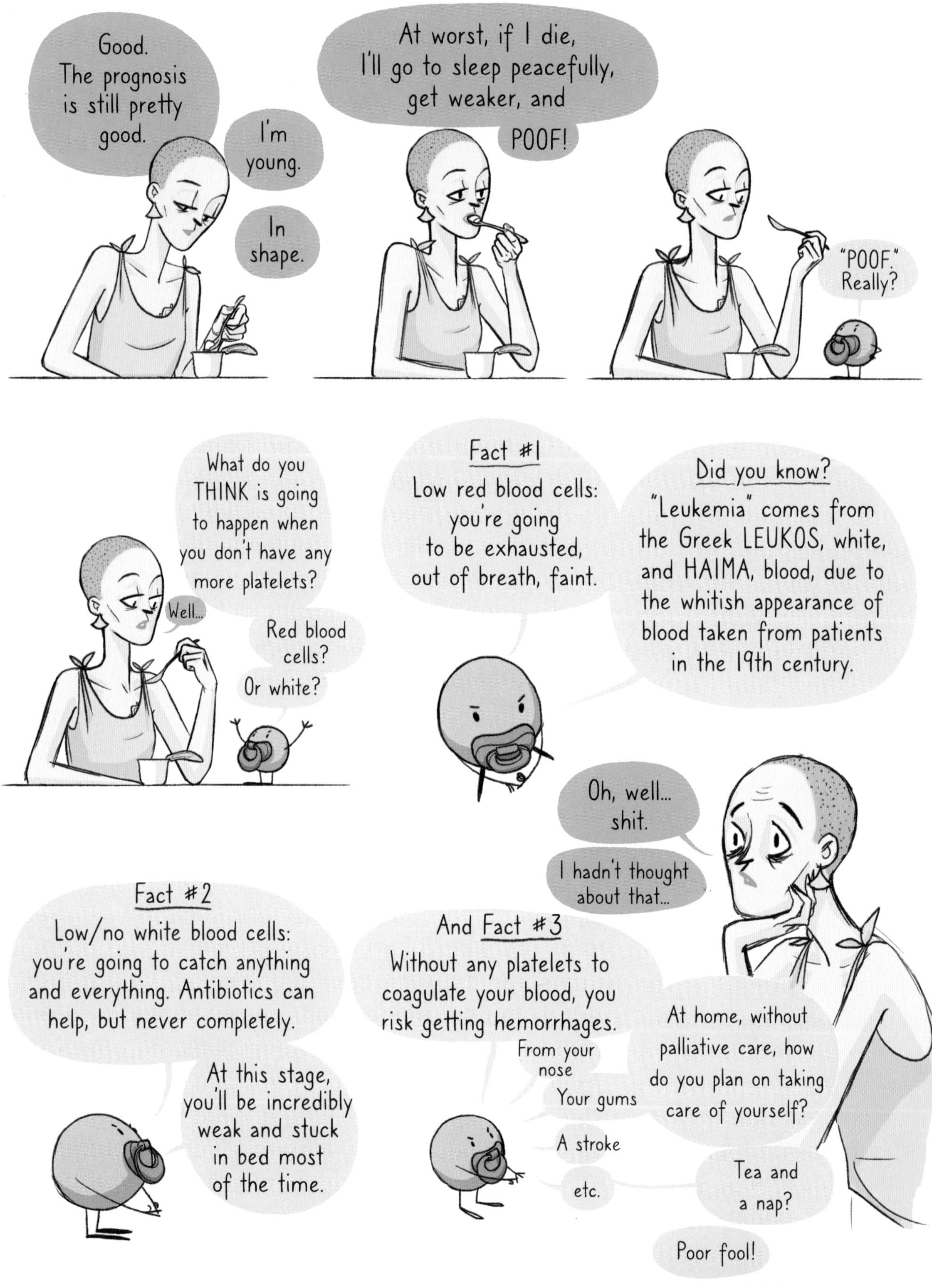

Good. The prognosis is still pretty good.

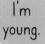

I'm young.

In shape.

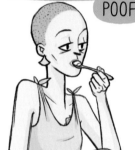

At worst, if I die, I'll go to sleep peacefully, get weaker, and POOF!

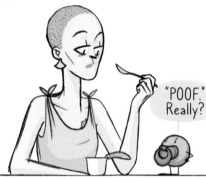

"POOF." Really?

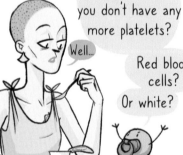

What do you THINK is going to happen when you don't have any more platelets?

Well...

Red blood cells?

Or white?

Fact #1
Low red blood cells: you're going to be exhausted, out of breath, faint.

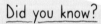

Did you know?
"Leukemia" comes from the Greek LEUKOS, white, and HAIMA, blood, due to the whitish appearance of blood taken from patients in the 19th century.

Oh, well... shit.

I hadn't thought about that...

Fact #2
Low/no white blood cells: you're going to catch anything and everything. Antibiotics can help, but never completely.

At this stage, you'll be incredibly weak and stuck in bed most of the time.

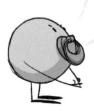

And Fact #3
Without any platelets to coagulate your blood, you risk getting hemorrhages.
From your nose
Your gums
A stroke
etc.

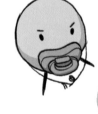

At home, without palliative care, how do you plan on taking care of yourself?

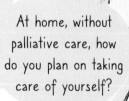

Tea and a nap?

Poor fool!

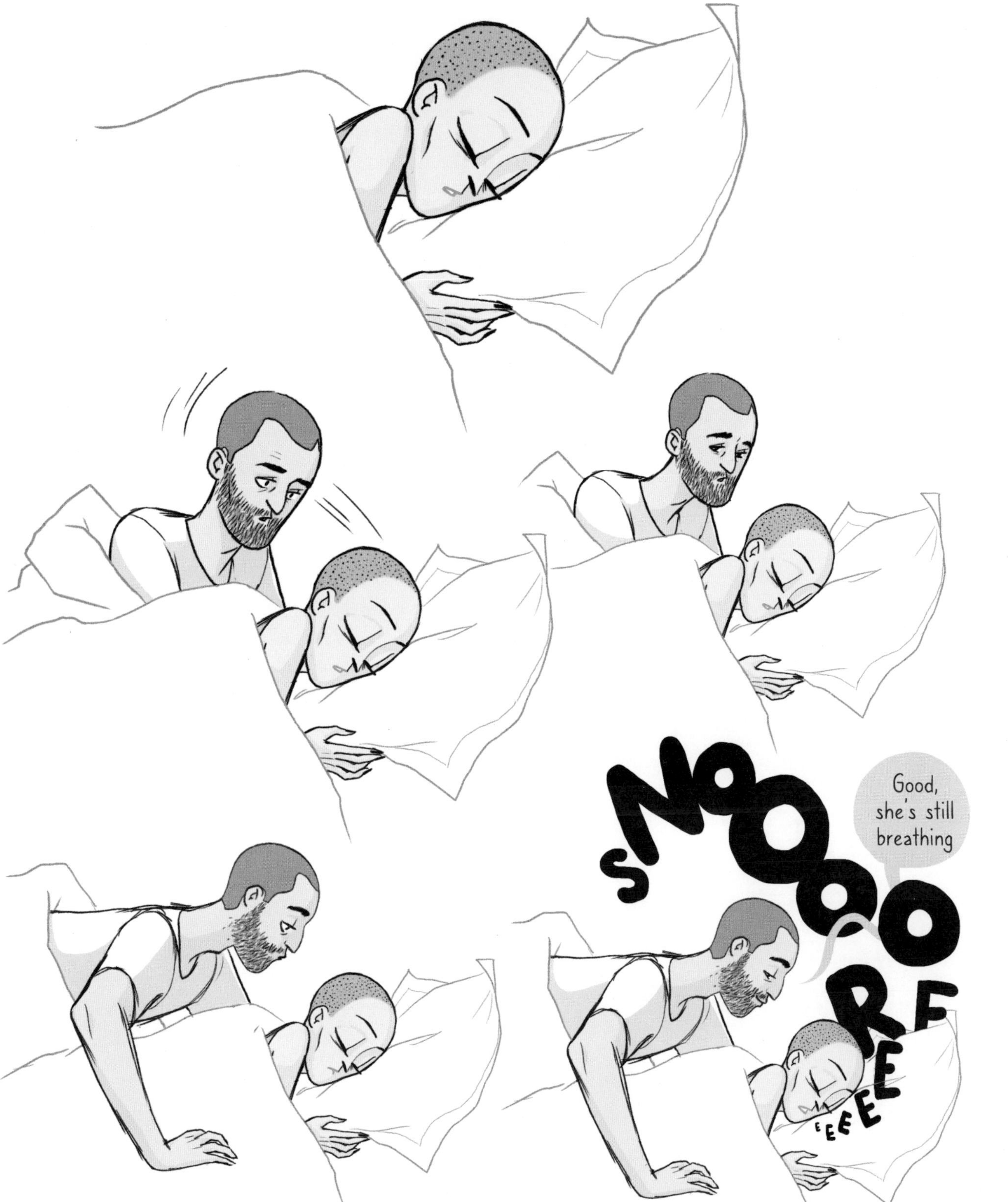
SNOOOORFEEEEE
Good, she's still breathing

Catherine drew her last breath on July 31, 2017.

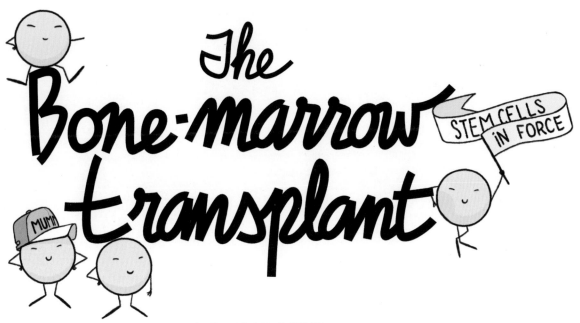

The Bone-marrow transplant

STEM CELLS IN FORCE

BACKGROUND

Bone marrow is a spongy tissue found in the hollow part of bones. It contains hematopoietic stem cells (HSC). These become white blood cells, red blood cells, and platelets.

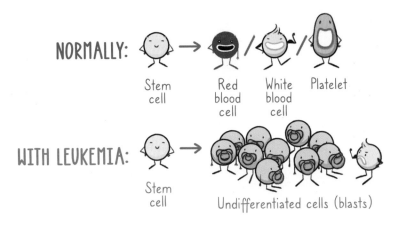

NORMALLY:

Stem cell → Red blood cell / White blood cell / Platelet

WITH LEUKEMIA:

Stem cell → Undifferentiated cells (blasts)

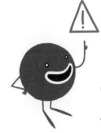

⚠️ There's no bone marrow in the spinal cord, which is instead made up of nerves.

WHEN IT'S TIME...

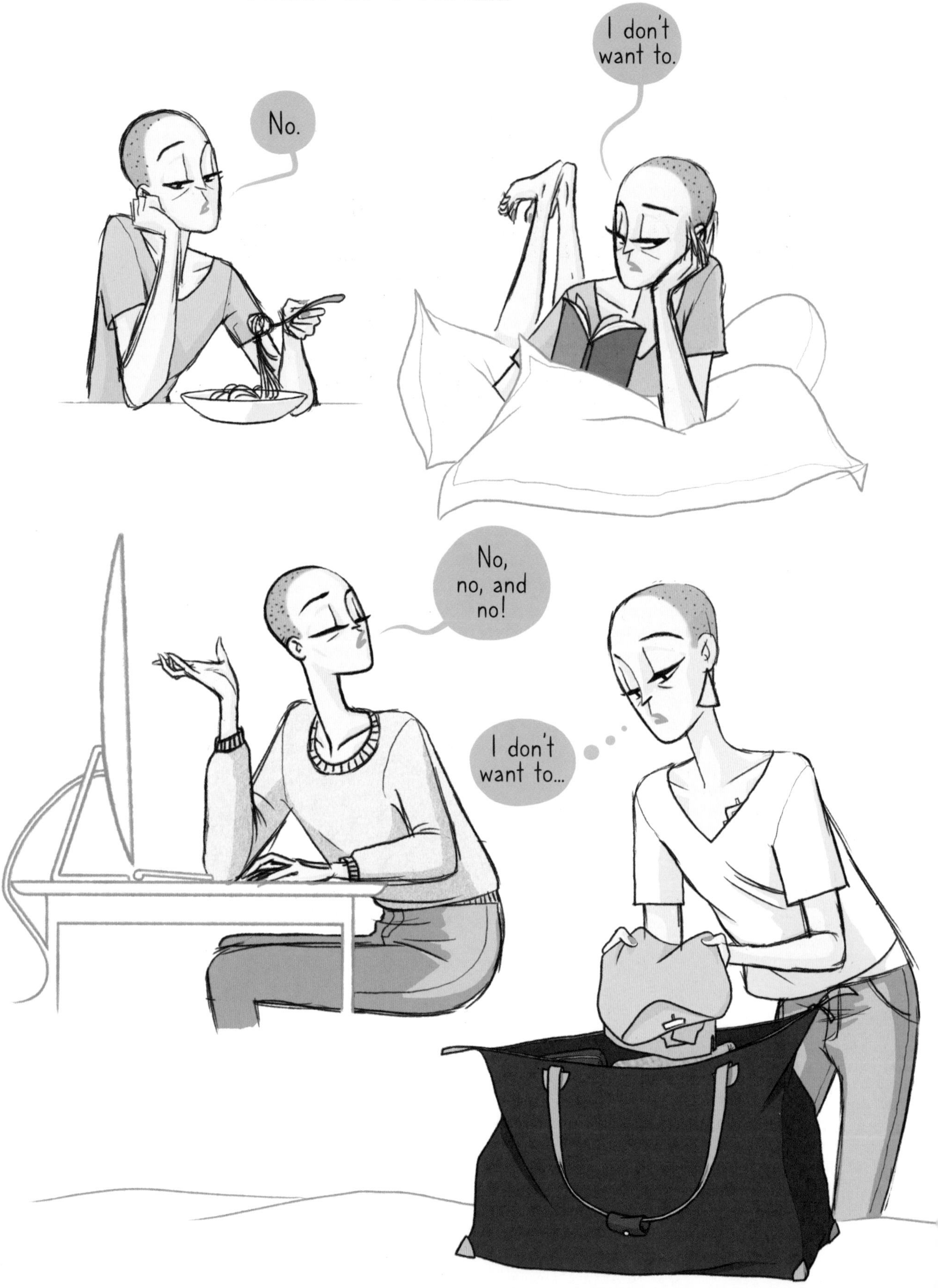
No.
I don't want to.
No, no, and no!
I don't want to...

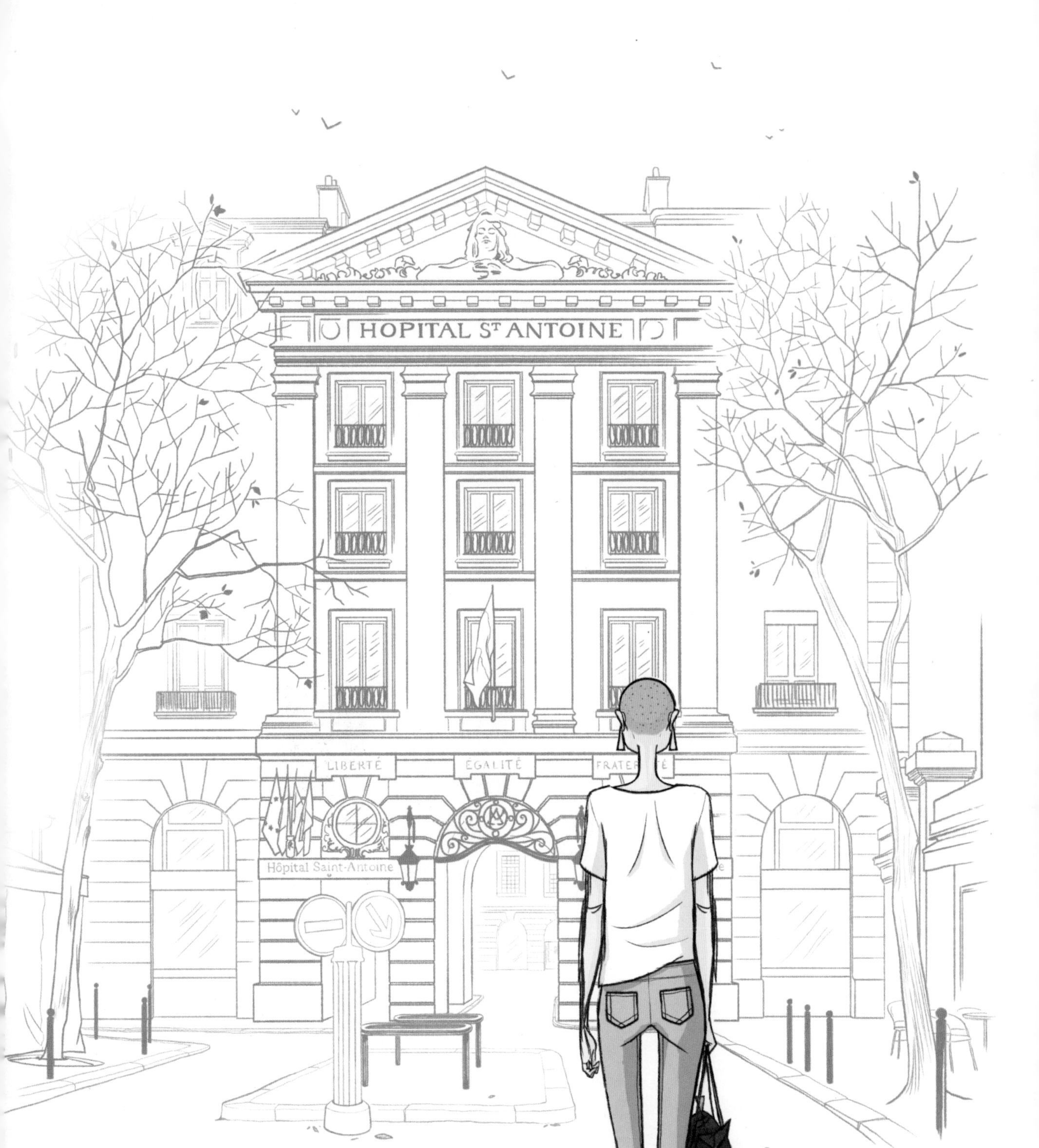
HOPITAL St ANTOINE
LIBERTÉ
ÉGALITÉ
Hôpital Saint-Antoine
JUNE 26, 2015
No 4th chemo, as it happens. We're going straight to a bone marrow transplant.
I don't want to go in there...

WHEN IT'S TIME...

With time passing and my cell count increasing too slowly,
there's no 4th consolidation chemo. The time for the **TRANSPLANT** has come!

I'm going to be hospitalized for more than a month,
and I'm well prepared.

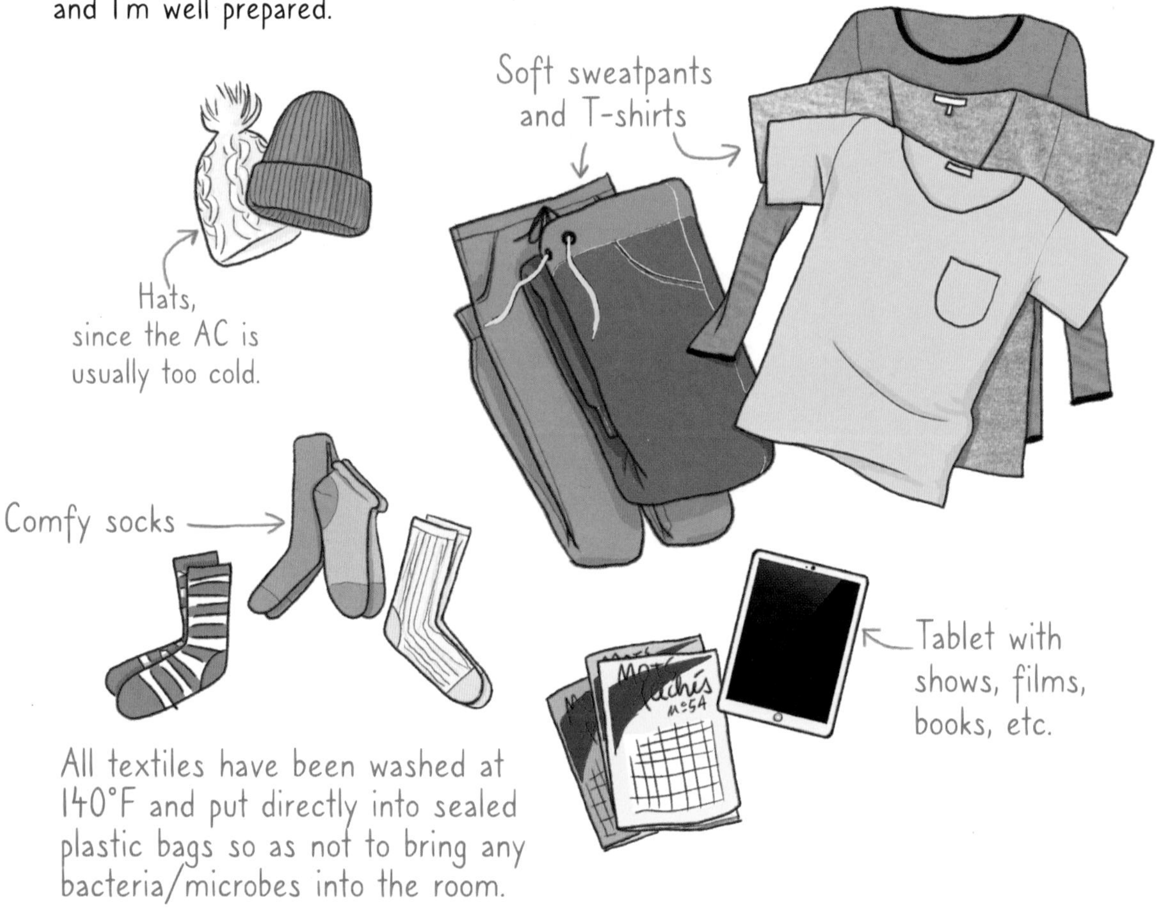
Soft sweatpants and T-shirts
Hats, since the AC is usually too cold.
Comfy socks
Tablet with shows, films, books, etc.
All textiles have been washed at 140°F and put directly into sealed plastic bags so as not to bring any bacteria/microbes into the room.

We're starting with a **CONDITIONING** phase.
It consists of 7 days of intense chemo, in order
to prepare my body to receive the transplant.

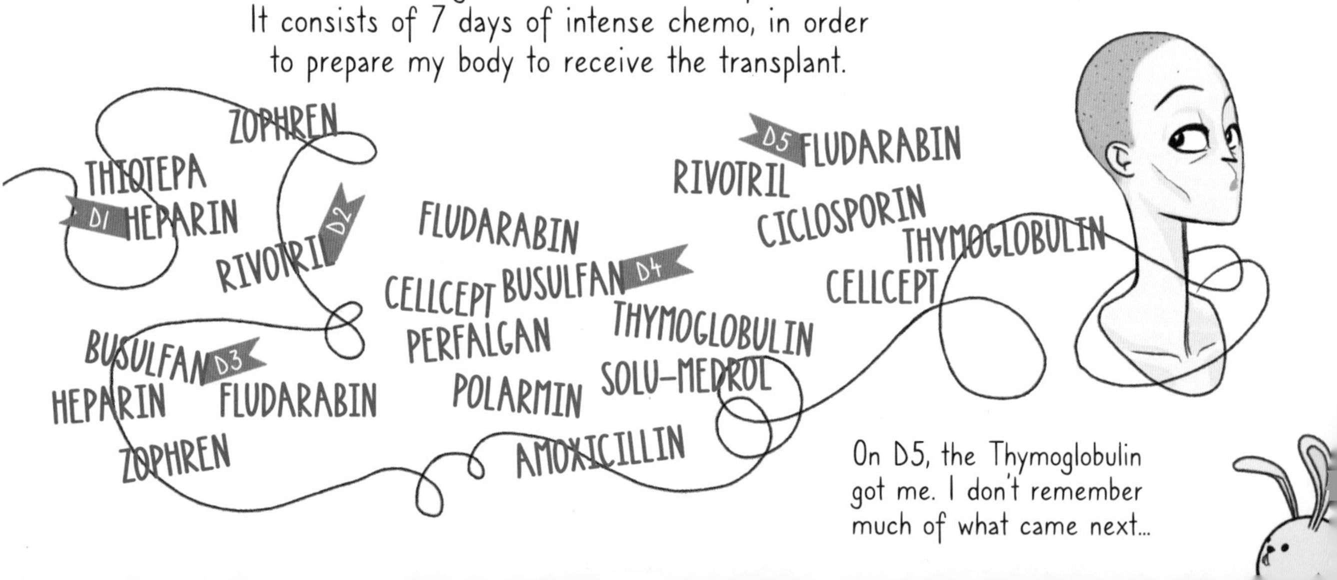
ZOPHREN
THIOTEPA
D1 HEPARIN
D2
RIVOTRIL
FLUDARABIN
CELLCEPT BUSULFAN D4
PERFALGAN
THYMOGLOBULIN
BUSULFAN D3
HEPARIN FLUDARABIN
POLARMIN
SOLU-MEDROL
ZOPHREN
AMOXICILLIN
D5 FLUDARABIN
RIVOTRIL
CICLOSPORIN
THYMOGLOBULIN
CELLCEPT

On D5, the Thymoglobulin
got me. I don't remember
much of what came next...

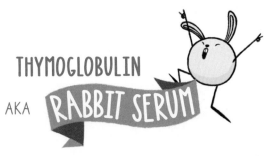

THYMOGLOBULIN

AKA RABBIT SERUM

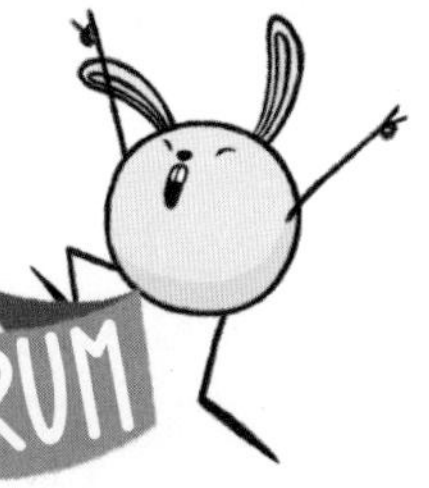

An anti-lymphocyte serum made from **RABBIT** proteins and human lymphocytes.
ITS GOAL: fight against transplant rejections.
DURATION: about 20 hours.
Every 15 minutes, my vitals are taken (blood pressure, oxygenation, heartbeat, and temperature), then every half hour.

For **20 HOURS. DAY AND NIGHT.**

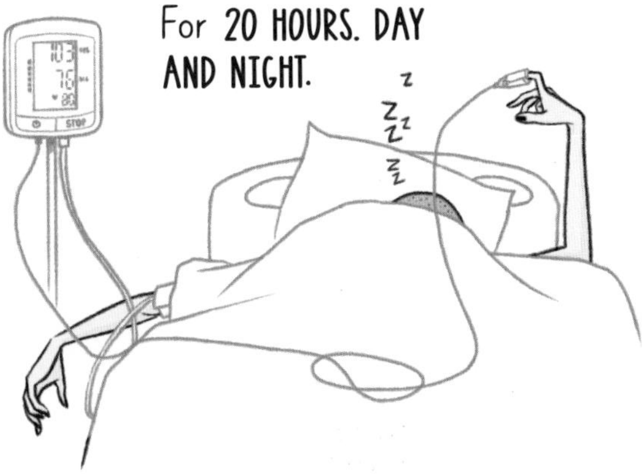

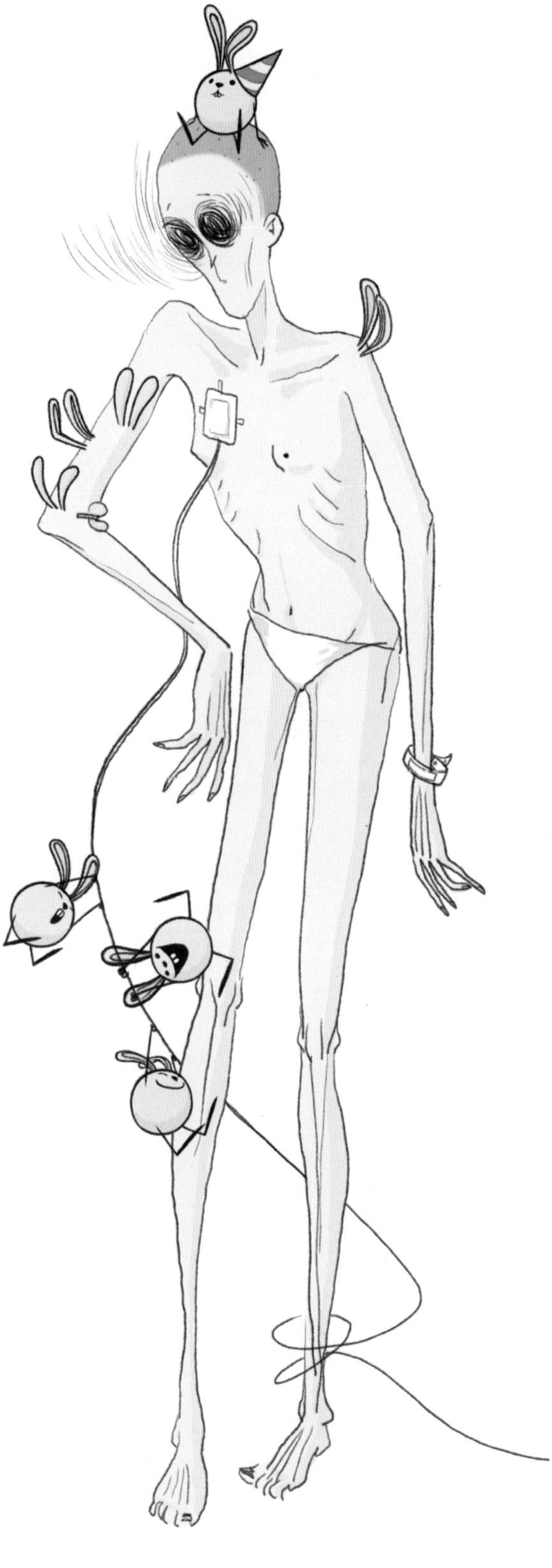

SIDE EFFECTS: It's a **TRIP**. My head turns into rabbit soup. Sometimes I'm in control but most of the time I'm completely out of it. I have some insane dreams, and I can't remember where I am or even my own name.

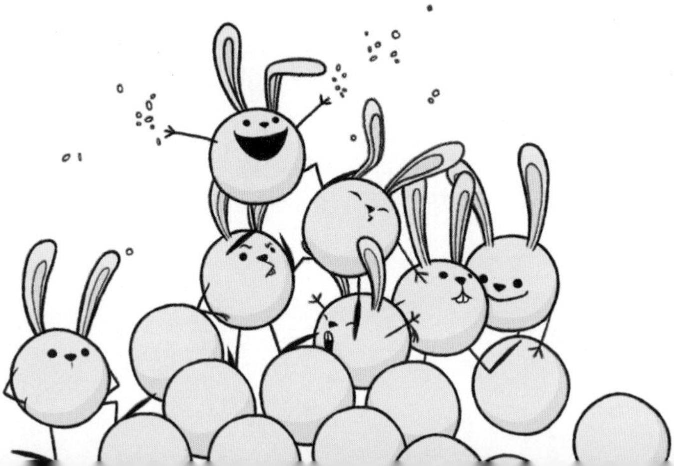

D-DAY

Here it is, here we are... Gabriel donated his stem cells a few days earlier. He joins me in my room. It's scary. It's like the lottery: so long as you haven't checked the numbers, you might be a millionaire. So long as I haven't had the transplant, I might be cured. The uncertainty is comforting.

It's 6:00 in the evening.

In that moment, <u>all my bone marrow is gone.</u> It's been completely fried by the chemo to prepare for the transplant.

It looks like raw meat. Drab pink.

It's strange.

Like I'm missing an organ.

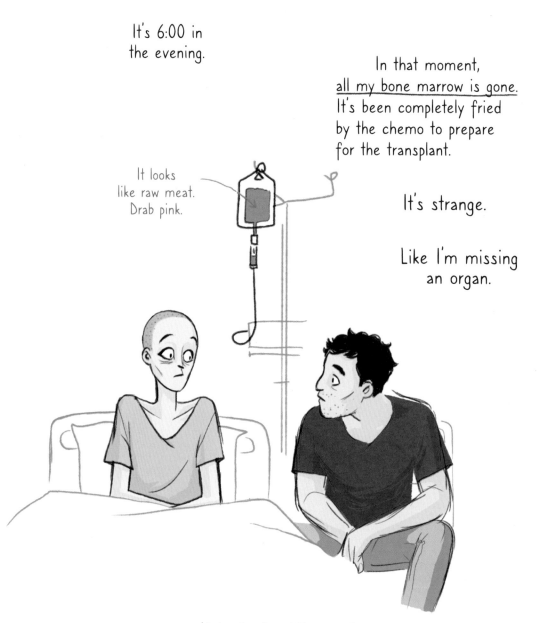

It lasts for 15 minutes.

It's over.

D+1 Now, we wait.
If a bacterium, a fever, or whatever turns up, it'll be dealt with.
Waiting around with nothing to do is the worst.

D+2 I'm fed with a nasogastric tube because I'm probably going to get **MUCOSITIS** (ulcers in the mouth—I mean a LOT, making it impossible to eat).

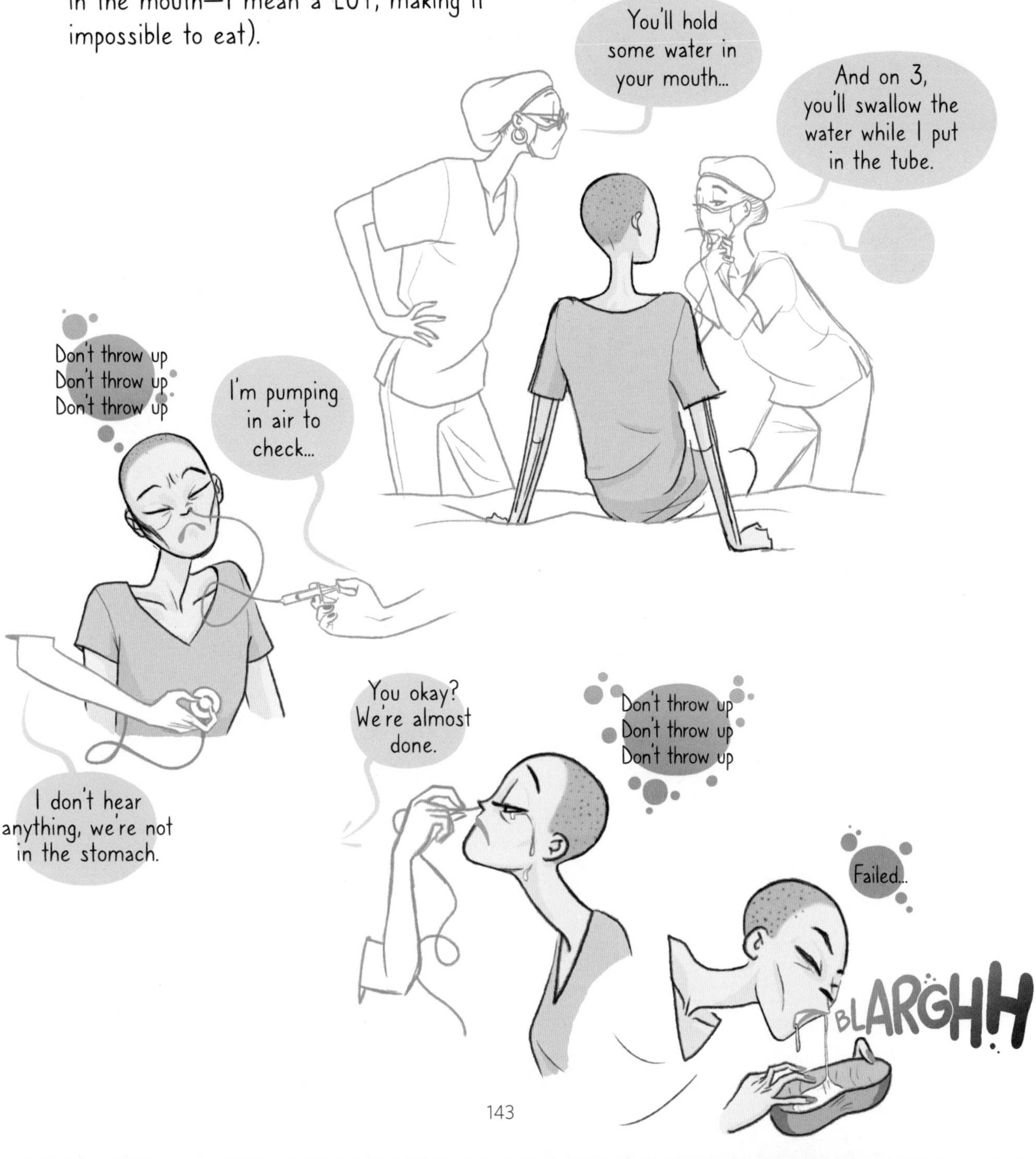

You'll hold some water in your mouth...
And on 3, you'll swallow the water while I put in the tube.
Don't throw up
Don't throw up
Don't throw up
I'm pumping in air to check...
I don't hear anything, we're not in the stomach.
You okay? We're almost done.
Don't throw up
Don't throw up
Don't throw up
Failed...
BLARGHH

GIVING MARROW

All the cells in our body have, on their surface, molecules called HLA ("human leukocyte antigens"). These are their ID cards. Our white blood cells know these molecules, and if they encounter cells that don't have the right HLA combination, they destroy them. This is what happens to microbes and bacteria that are destroyed, most of the time, before they make us sick.

WTF
ABC

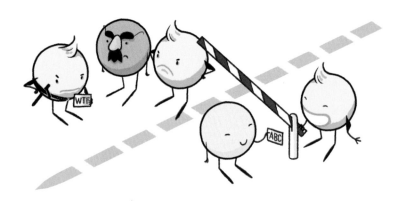

Thus, for a bone marrow transplant, you have to find a donor whose HLA type is the closest possible to the recipient's, so that the recipient's antibodies don't destroy the transplant. With brothers and sisters, there's a 1 in 4 chance of finding a donor (25%, pretty low!). But sometimes, even in a group of 8, no one is compatible. In that case, you have to find a volunteer donor in the international registry (40% chance of finding one).

HLA HLA
HLA HLA
Father
Mother
HLA HLA
HLA HLA
HLA HLA
HLA HLA
Recipient
Compatible donor

As far as donors go, a Caucasian won't be compatible with an Asian or an African, since the HLA molecules are too different. And finding a compatible donor when you're of mixed race is even more complicated, as you have to find someone with the same "mix."

So if you're half Indian, half Russian?
Turkish/Korean?
Malagasy/Chinese?
Thai, Gabonese?
Brazilian/Inuit?
Sioux/German?
Swedish, Tamil?
That would be tricky.

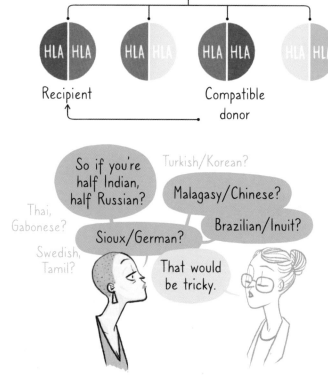

So it's really important that people sign up for a volunteer registry in order for there to be the largest selection of potential donors as possible (e.g., at www.bethematch.org).

There are 2 ways to harvest marrow. APHERESIS is a nonsurgical method where peripheral blood stem cells (PBSC) are extracted from the bloodstream. ASPIRATION is a surgical method where liquid marrow containing the body's stem cells is withdrawn from both sides of the back of the pelvic bone.

HOW DOES DONATION WORK?

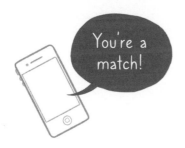

A patient needs a transplant, and you're a match! The donation center decides on the date of the extraction.

You participate in an information session, where you learn about the procedure and recovery process, including risks and side effects. ✓

You sign a consent form. ✓

You have a physical exam and give blood samples to make sure that the donation will be safe for both you and the recipient. ✓

OPTION #1: APHERESIS, OR PBSC DONATION
(at a blood center or outpatient facility)

For five days prior to the donation, you'll receive injections of a medication that increases the number of stem cells in your bloodstream.

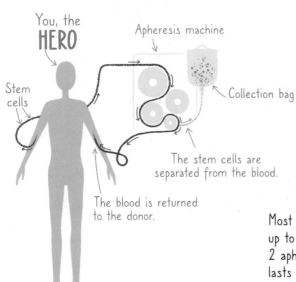

You, the HERO

Apheresis machine

Collection bag

Stem cells

The stem cells are separated from the blood.

The blood is returned to the donor.

GOOD TO KNOW

You may experience headaches or bone or muscle aches from the injections you receive prior to the donation. Most donors report a full recovery within 7-10 days of donation.

Most PBSC donations are completed in one session lasting up to 8 hours. In some cases, donations are completed in 2 apharesis sessions lasting 4-6 hours each. The process lasts about 4 hours, and if not enough stem cells are drawn, then zip! A second 4-hour session! This type of drawing is painless (besides the shots in the buttocks and the drips).

OPTION #2: ASPIRATION
(in the hospital)

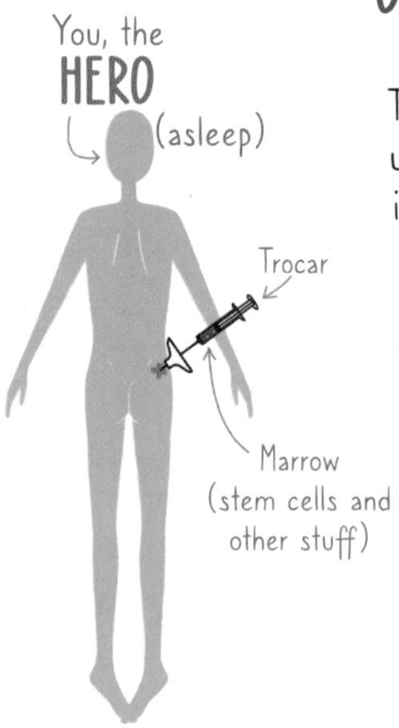

This extraction method requires hospitalization. It happens under general anesthesia and in an operating room, and there is no risk of paralysis (contrary to certain popular myths).

In this case, there are no injections beforehand to get stem cells into the bloodstream, since they're going directly to the source.

You, the
HERO
(asleep)

Trocar

Marrow
(stem cells and
other stuff)

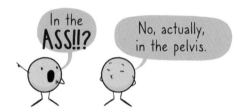

In the
ASS!!?

No, actually,
in the pelvis.

AFTER THE DONATION

Typical side effects of marrow donation can include back or hip pain, throat pain, muscle pain, fatigue, insomnia, headache, dizziness, loss of appetite, and nausea. Full recovery takes about 20 days, and you will be monitored until you report a full recovery.

But in any case,

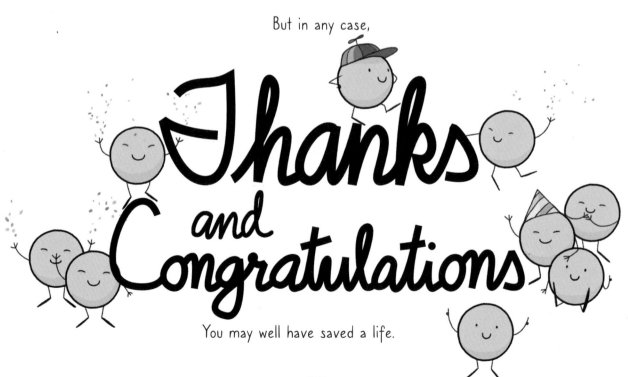

Thanks
and
Congratulations

You may well have saved a life.